LET'S TALK
TANTRA

**WITH ULRIK ADINATHA LYSHØJ
BY LOTTE SØS FARRAN-LEE**

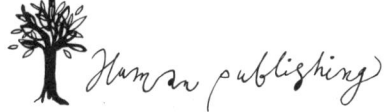

Let's Talk Tantra #1 Book in the series Let's Talk © Human Publishing at Let's Talk series .

© Lotte Søs FarranLee & Ulrik Adinatha Lyshøj 2017

Lotte Søs FarranLee & Ulrik Adinatha Lyshøj have the rights as authors of this book.

All rights reserved, including the right to reproduce this book or portions thereof in any form whatsoever, without prior permission from the publisher except for short quotations used in reviews. The material contained in this book is for reference purposes only, and is not intended as a substitute for counselling, or other medical and/or therapeutic services.

1. edition 1. print 2017

Photos: Shutterstock

isbn 9788799843046

Published by
Human Publishing Worldwide ApS
www.humanpublishing.com
Email: info@humanpublishing.com

Contents

About Let's Talk, by Lotte Søs Farran-Lee
About Ulrik Adinatha Lyshøj

Chapter 1: Why do we talk about tantra?
Chapter 2: What is tantra?
Chapter 3: Tantra and the whole human being
Chapter 4: The tools of tantra
Chapter 5: Tantra on the individual plane
Chapter 6: The man and the woman
Chapter 7: You, me and tantra
Chapter 8: Tantra's goal and wrapping up

About the Tantra Temple
About Let's Talk series

Why – Let's Talk tantra?

First and foremost I wish to create, from deep inside of my heart, and share what my heart is full of, with the world.

When the series Let's Talk was ready to be created and the list of possible subjects was infinite… why did I then choose to start with tantra?

Tantra has a very special place in my heart. It has helped me through a spontaneous and intense spiritual awakening, also named Kundalini. Through the healing of the Kundalini, tantra crossed my path, and it became a long and beautiful journey leading back to myself.

The tantric love, the love for myself, the love for others and for the world became the reason for this to become the first book. I wanted the world to see the depth of tantric philosophy and why tantra is much more than just good sex, as it is so often presented. It is also an often widely misunderstood subject and the interpretations of what tantra is are many; therefore I wanted to create a conversation where I knew that the deep roots of tantra and philosophy came to light in an simple and grounded way.

I have known Ulrik Adinatha for many years and choosing him for my interview, was a very easy choice. Ulrik has a deeprooted understanding of tantra, and many years of practice. He has indeed shown to be an eligible contributor.

The conversation flowed very easily and we feel confident that tantra has gotten its due space in a simple and respectful way.

I'm delighted to share the first Let's Talk book with you.

Love
Lotte Søs FarranLee
Author

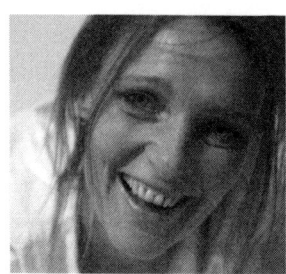

About Ulrik Adinatha Lyshøj, coauthor.
Tantra teacher, tantra masseur, leader and cofounder of the Tantra Temple in Denmark.

Ulrik Adinatha has since the year 2000 been on a very deep and honest journey exploring himself and tantra. He has a wish to help others on their spiritual journey and to show people the essence of tantra, to help them open their hearts and let love show the way.

It was not an obvious choice for him to walk the tantric path, this farm boy who grew up in the countryside in a tranquil family setting. However, already at a very young age, a quest to become the perfect lover and the wish to be able to communicate and teach it to others appeared.

His quest to become the perfect lover led him into the tantric world – a world that fully embraced that quest. In the essence of tantra, he also found the possibility to raise sexuality to a completely different level through the heart. Along the way, he found that tantra had so much more to offer – the possibility to become a more whole person. Tantra is a practice of continuous transformation; everything he communicates in this book is an expression of the ideal human being that he aims to become.

Ulrik Adinatha embodies and passes on the tantric philosophy with great integrity in the tantric practice. It is his deepest wish that more and more people will discover the way to the love within themselves, and through that experience give more pure love to themselves, their loved ones and people in general by the tantric practice.

He is a pioneer in the tantric world in Denmark and is deeply anchored in the tantric philosophy and tantric practice.

Ulrik Adinatha is passing his knowledge on through teaching, tantric massages, workshops, talks and his daily work as a leader of the Tantra Temple in Denmark.

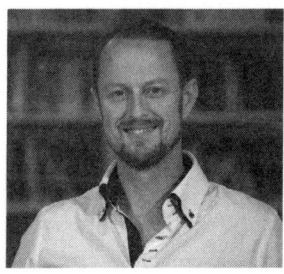

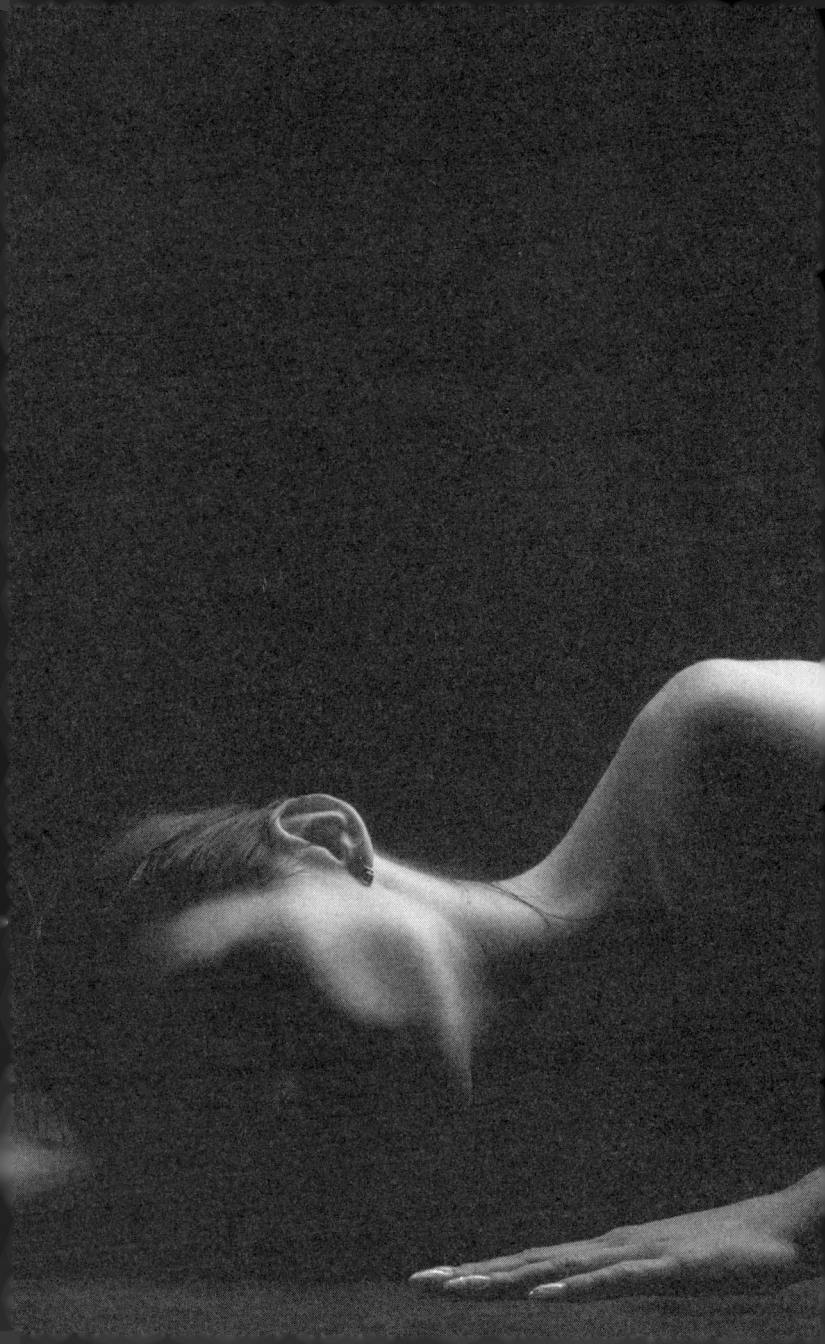

CHAPTER 1:
Why should we talk about Tantra?

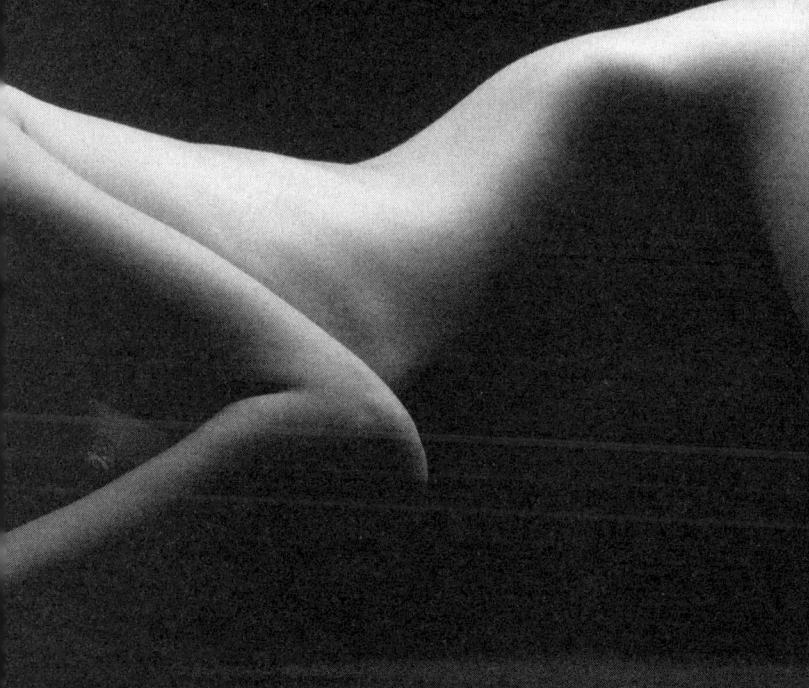

Why should we talk about Tantra?

Because it is important! Because tantra is a science of life, about living our life, dealing the most material aspects to the most spiritual dimensions.

It's a life science, which has been handed over from one to another for thousands of years. And even though our culture and society has changed dramatically throughout the years… we're still just human beings. There are still some basic structures and principles about being a human being. We are still the same within and tantra continues to have the answers to all the small and big questions in life, and all the solutions to the many problems we human beings struggle with.

Tantra fits into every place in life, therefore I think it is important – everybody can benefit from tantra. Wherever and whenever. Tantra offers a greater understanding of ourselves as humans and thus we are able to get much more out of life.

Tantra is notoriously known for its approach to human sexuality, because it has such an open approach to it. Tantra says: "Instead of hiding it away, let us use the sexuality to enhance our lives in all aspects". Tantra is pertinent to all aspects of our lives and not only the sexual, despite the common focus on just that particular area.

Another reason it is so interesting to talk about tantra is the fact that sexuality still appears to be quite forbidden. By talking about it we can open up and allow it to become an integrated part of our emotional lives, rather than being unable to feel our own sexuality and hence feeling cut off from part of ourselves. So talking about tantra helps us become more connected with ourselves – also through our sexual energy.

Sexuality is important to all of us, whether it is present or missing. This is so because sexuality is the strongest energy we have. With this energy we are able to create life. Man and woman in unison have the power to create new life with it. Through tantra we are able to make use of the potency of this energy in other areas of our life.

We can transform it into other energies, and thereby consciously make use of the sexual energy in all areas of our life – our work life, spiritual life, and ability to stay focused and present – yes, basically everything that we do in life.

If we learn how to use it, learn how to master the sexual energy, we can then use it actively. We should tame it, not suppress it, but rather control it. So that we are capable of actively and consciously choosing how we will use it.

At the same time we have to bring the other aspects of life into our sexuality, so that we naturally carry our emotions with us. It will then become completely natural; that it is love that connects us when we are with another person, and not only desire. It then becomes love that connects one human to another. A deep wish from one soul to another soul to become one. At that moment we are not only having a sexual experience, which is based on lust, friction and orgasm. Then it becomes a tantric meeting of lovemaking, a meeting between two souls wishing to connect deeply with each other at all levels.

It is also interesting to talk about tantra because tantra helps us become not only creators of our life, but also conscious creators of our life and thereby able to enable each other to become more true to what we already are.

It is important to talk about sexuality because it is what people associate with tantra, but it is also quite relevant to talk about all the other aspects of tantra, and thereby sowing seeds of understanding that tantra is not just about sexuality, but about the all of life. That it is indeed a very diverse life philosophy.

What will the reader get out of this conversation?

The philosophy of tantra can help the reader become more conscious about themselves and their life in general.

Help us open up to the fact that we do have a conscious choice here in life. Many people live a life where they don't feel that they are free. Tantra can help them to feel free at all levels. We are never trapped in a marriage or a work situation. We always have all possibilities in front of us and we can choose what is best for us – for our own spiritual journey right now.

Often we make choices based on the values we have been raised with or what society tells us, or what we think is the most logical or reasonable. We often choose the job that pays the highest salary, or the girl or boyfriend that is the most beautiful, or the one that has the potential to become the best dad or mom to our children. The mental checklist tells us what looks the best on paper. Many studies show that people don't become happier by having more money, but still many people think that a bigger car, house or flat screen TV will make them happier. Tantra helps us find the true source of happiness within us. It is this source that is our connection to our soul; that often has a completely different mission or journey than our rational mind tells us.

It could be that it would be much more satisfying for our soul to work as a volunteer and just make enough to make ends meet than to work in a highly paid job. I don't claim that this is true for all readers. But we have to let go of the idea of how things should be and instead use our heart and listen to that inner voice that knows so well why we are here.

You can choose tantra because it is a system with which you completely openly and honestly can analyse yourself and find out how you can grow, and you can start just where you are right now in your life. It is not like other spiritual paths or religions where you have to do something special or be something special to get there. In tantra you begin just where you are in your life, and then you use that place as a starting point. Whether it is about healing something within yourself, or enjoying a better sex life, or the wish to surrender to your own spiritual journey.

Tantra provides you with all the tools to analyse where you are right now, and all the tools to become an even better version of yourself. It enables you to change all the traits you would like to change or expand all good qualities you may discover on the way, that you have not fully awakened yet. Tantra works with the areas of human qualities that are still only seeds – something that has not yet developed – and something that this person would have a natural talent for, if he or she were just looking in that direction. This process is called transfiguration, which is the ability to see beyond the immediate. With the help of our intuition it enables us to sense some of those qualities that are not yet developed in ourselves, in others, in a situation or in a phenomenon. It encourages that specific ability or quality consciously and helps us to evolve ourselves or others around us. It is most powerful in relation to the people we love and through this process one can really achieve great progress.

What is tantra not?

Tantra is experiencing a period of heightened attention and it has become an "inword". Many people who are drawn towards it decide to attend a weekend seminar or workshop and then following they decide that they want to teach it themselves. "I would like to pass this on to other people, write a book or make a movie about it." They then mix it with a bit of this and a bit of that of what they already know and then call it tantra. Often they have not understood how profound it actually is and they have not understood that it is a science about the whole human being and so much more than just the sexuality.

When we are talking about tantric massage, which is a popular way to experience tantra, I have encountered many people, who have none or a quite limited level of education and who call themselves tantra masseurs. They may have taken a few seminars or a short education or maybe they have seen some videos. Then they have decided "I can do that", without even knowing the deeper perspective. It is often this which makes tantra misunderstood, because the deeper perspective is lacking.

At the Tantra Temple we are very aware that we need to work on our own lives before we are able to help other people make changes in their lives. If we would like to work with the energies of other people, it requires us to have a very intimate understanding of our own energy and a deep personal practice first. But our society and culture does not allow the time to acquire that deep practice, which is the reason that tantra has become so misunderstood and diluted.

There are many who think that tantra is just good sex. Then they learn some tantric techniques and then they mix it to a sexuality seminar, where they use some of them. If some of the tantric techniques prove to be too difficult or too advanced and therefore "unsellable", they are left out. They sell the parts of tantra that they think people will find interesting, and aim to get as many as possible to attend the seminar or to sell the most books, so that they will have a good business. This means that the philosophy about the whole human being, and the idea of the erotic starting from the heart, and that there has to be a deep love between the two, are all too difficult. It all takes too long, so "let's cut that out", but then it is no longer tantra.

In tantra you strive to get to the point where you don't lose the energy via ejaculations or explosive orgasms. For some this is too difficult. That is why some of the tantric techniques that focus on getting a stronger and longer lasting erection, and on how to enjoy the most fantastic orgasms – are exactly the techniques they keep. But the abstinence from ejaculations is much too challenging. Too many men would not go into this work or they would assume that it is too difficult – therefore they just teach them how to hold their erection longer before ejaculating in the end. But that is exactly why tantra enters a grey zone because this is not tantra.

Tantra does not compromise, tantra goes all the way.

Tantra is explained in many and various ways and because tantra massage is a very intimate and sensual massage, there exists a grey zone between serious tantra massage and prostitution.

Some tantra masseurs feel this way: "If I give my guest a good experience and if I like them and they like me and we're open about for it, then we can also have sex together". It might feel right in the moment but it is very easy to lose the focus, which should be to initiate the other person in tantra and help them gain a deeper understanding of themselves.

The assumption that the masseur does it for their own desire and just want to be with a lot of women is one of the classic misunderstandings about tantra. That might be true in some cases, but then is it not tantra?

In the work field of massage, touch or therapy, you are bound to come across people who touch other human beings for their own sake, because they themselves like it. Any man who enjoys touching naked women has it made for himself if he is able to present it as a service and a paying job.

Others perform the massage for the sake of the recipients' egos, to give them something he or she likes, a feeling of being good, useful, loved or whatever it might be.

But in a true tantric meeting you touch without ego. You offer yourself as a channel for whatever might pass through you – at that exact moment. At times, it might be something that the other person didn't know he or she needed and yet it might be the right thing to do at that moment to facilitate the change for the person you work with. You tune into a higher flow and say: "Now I am opening myself up as a channel to give that other person what he/she needs right now". It might be something quite different from what that person expected beforehand, but preferences or expectations are not the focus of the tantric meeting.

What are some common reservations about tantra?

Some of the reservations that I hear are: "Tantra is all about group sex" or "Tantra has to do with free sex" or "In tantra you engage in sex with anyone". Others say that tantra is much too spiritual for them or that tantra requires you to behave in a certain way, or that you need to walk around with a bindi on your forehead, wear chakra clothes or be this kind of hippie newage person. There are some very rigid perceptions about how and what it is.

What are people afraid of?

They think tantra massage is sex and that it is something sexual, a sexual service, that you purchase. That it is just prostitution in a pretty disguise.

This is a very common reason why people are nervous. In addition, some people fear being fully open to themselves and to live their life to the fullest. There is a fear of meeting oneself and facing the truths one might prefer to be ignorant of.

Tantra gives you the tools to look at yourself and see yourself exactly as you are at this very moment, with both the good things and the bad things.

Tantra also gives you the tools to make changes. But it requires a tremendous amount of honesty and that honesty can be very difficult to achieve if you have been used to living a life of lies. If you have lied to yourself and others about who you really are. Once you open up to it, tantra has the ability to act as a mirror of your true self, and this can cause a great deal of anxiety.

The masseur and the guest do not know what will be unleashed during a massage. They do not know what they will experience, what shadows the guest hides in his/her subconscious, but they are encouraged to trust that they will get through it.

A professional masseur will progress at the speed the guest is ready for and will not open up to the next level until the guest is ready for it. The masseur does not wait for the guest to feel ready, this might never happen. He opens up to the next level once he senses with his empathy that the guest is ready.

Tantra massage is not a sexual service that you purchase and where you can place an order, like: "I would like to have those multiorgasms." But together with the masseur you can find areas that you would like to work with, and through this work you will experience brand new parts of yourself. But it is not something which can be ordered. It will always be the assessment of the masseur.

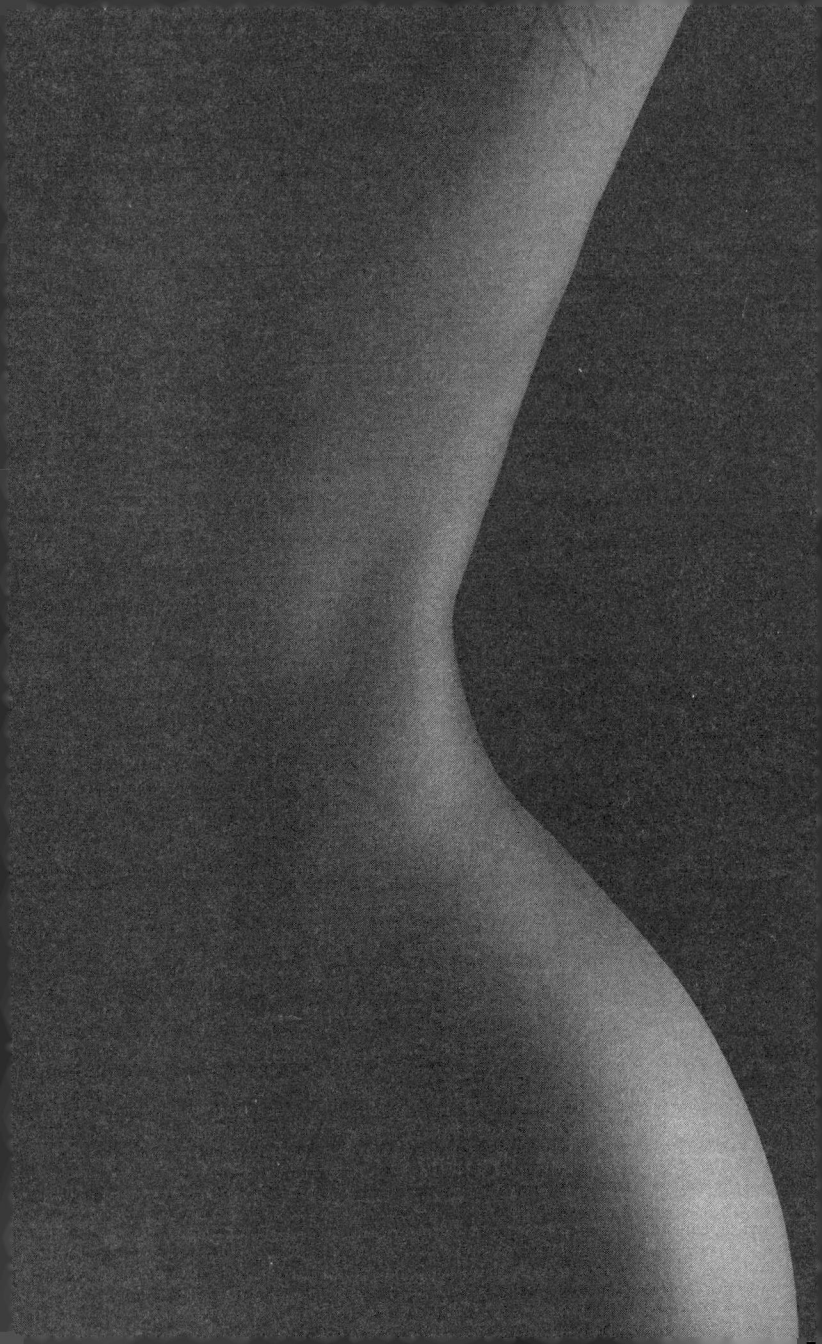

CHAPTER 2:
What is tantra?

What is tantra?

Tantra is a way of living. It is life itself. It is to be able to encompass the whole human life, without inhibitions, no taboos, no limitations and to learn how we can use everything which we as humans have been given to empower our own growth and spiritual journey and return home as spiritual beings.

Tantra is surrounded by a lot of mystery and misunderstanding. Ultimately it can only be understood by living it and not by talking, writing or reading about it.

It can be used to awaken a curiosity and interest, and it can be used to remind people on a deeper level that they are so much more than what they believe to they are. That they are much greater and part of something much larger. In this way tantra can create a way for people to begin exploring themselves as whole, living human beings and spiritual creatures, because only then are we really able to understand what tantra is.

A traditional saying goes, "You have to taste the honey to know the honey". If people never tasted honey… no writing or reading about it would make them understand what honey really is.

When talking or writing about tantra, it is with the purpose of awakening people, so that they may be able to take the first baby steps towards an understanding of themselves and of tantra.

Sometimes tantra is also called "to be walking on the edge of a knife". The true tantric way is so narrow and delicate that you can easily fall off. You just lose balance and then you will fall off the true spiritual path. This makes tantra "dangerous", because you can get lost so easily.

If you want to choose a spiritual system that will get you home safe; you should not choose tantra. Tantra is not a safe system. There are many other systems that can do that and that have set up numerous roadblocks to keep you on the right path. It is like walking in a valley: If you just continue straight forward you will eventually get there. Whereas with tantra you walk on the edge of a knife, and there is absolutely nothing keeping you from falling off the edge. It is important to remain focused on everything you do.

So it's a very active choice all the time?

Yes, all the time.

What is the philosophy in tantra?

There are basically four cornerstones of tantra: polarity, energy, love and transfiguration.

1. Polarity

The tantric way of working with energy is with the perspective that polarity is everywhere. It is the tension of dualistic opposites that produces energy.

The perfect symbol of this polarity is man and woman. It is no coincidence that we are born as two different sexes, with so much in common and yet so many differences that sets us apart.

If we look at the basics, then the greatest difference between man and woman is the genitals; designed so brilliantly that they fit perfectly together and at the same time become an expression of our polarity.

The male is extrovert; yang, firm and hard while the female is more introvert; yin, receptive, soft and open, and this is one of the polarities that is seen everywhere. However, this does not mean that the male is exclusively masculine and the female exclusively feminine, we all encompass both sides.

A strong and masculine man will be able to attract a very sensual feminine woman. Whereas a less masculine man? man will attract a less sensual woman and in such a relationship there is less energy. In a relationship with stronger polarity there will be much more energy present. Polarising the opposites is not only about sexes but also about energy.

In tantra we speak of Shiva, the masculine, and Shakti, the feminine, as archetypal symbols of the whole universal creation. Consciousness makes a plan and energy fills it out; together they create the whole universe. By understanding the polar interactions between the two and how they need to be in balance, we can make things happen and magically succeed. If there is more consciousness than energy, life will tend to be more dry, with good mental plans, but very little energy to fill it out and give it juice, power, life and nutrition.

Whereas if there is more energy than consciousness there will be more juice and power, but it will lack direction, without the consciousness. It will then be chaotic and very random, messy with a lot of energy pointing in all kinds of directions and nothing will ever be able to manifest. When the two are in balance, we are able to create magic, both on an individual level, in our relationships, in the meeting with the opposite sex, in our work relations, family, friends or where ever. We have our finger on the pulse and we are able judge if we need more energy or more consciousness, depending on the situation.

Our sexuality is a prime example of this. Here it becomes very obvious as the polarities are most obvious. Let us zoom in on our reproduction system, which is expressed at the sexual level. There we have one of the largest cells in the body, the female egg, which implants in the uterus and becomes the embryo and the symbol of energy. On the other hand we have one of the smallest cells in the human body, which is the sperm, which in reality is nothing more than a DNA package. But that DNA package contains a plan. It holds part of the plan of what this person is going to look like. The male sperm and the female egg unite and at that very moment we already have a plan for whom this new person will become and how he or she will develop.

If your relationship has become flat, boring, sluggish and without spark, it means that the polarity is not strong enough. With tantra it would be possible to consciously observe where it is missing and what needs to be done in order to change it. Not only to get the spark back, but to continuously keep the flame alive and be able to say to one another: "When we do this and this, then we experience the loss of energy, but when we do this and this, we awaken the flame and more consciousness and spark is present. Okay, let us avoid the things which depolarise us and focus on what creates a more powerful polarity". This way it is possible to develop the relationship instead of simply doing what feels familiar, cosy and safe.

It works the same way on the individual level. All the things you do, your wishes and aspirations, all the projects that you start, are about energy and consciousness. If you have a good plan, you need to empower it with a whole lot of juice and power. If you do not have a great plan, that is where to focus and improve while constantly working on obtaining the balance.

2. Energy

The second cornerstone is working with energy. It is about not wasting energy. We have a lot of energy available, but only when we are able to master the energy and work with it. To recirculate the energy and lift it to the highest possible level – and not release, exhaust, or excrete it.

Only at that point will we be able to use all that we have been given, and this is a very important part of the tantric philosophy.

At the sexual level it very obvious when the energy has been lost. Especially for the male. Because at the moment he ejaculates, he not only ejaculates the semen which holds many vitamins, minerals and nutrients, but he also loses a lot of energy. He is clearly more tired, exhausted and has less sexual desire, and he is often also less interested in intimacy afterwards, which is a clear sign that some of that energy, which was so intense before, is now lost.

From a human, physiological and spiritual perspective it is a waste to throw it all away. It is the best he can produce and it's all gone in one ejaculation. This is something which all spiritual traditions agree about, not only tantra: That it should not be wasted. How they choose to address this varies greatly. Most spiritual paths say "Let us avoid losing this energy, by just avoiding sexuality completely. Dry out the source and then give it all back to God."

But in regards to the sexual level, the tantric approach is more like: "Stop wasting the energy! Learn how to use it for much more than just pleasure."

It is not a quick fix though. We have to learn it all anew. Men tend to find this more difficult. The feeling of emptiness which stems from the release is in reality the natural male connection to the conscious aspect. The male nature is directed more towards the consciousness whereas the female nature is directed more towards the energy. This also shows in spiritual practice, where a more masculine practice is based on deep meditation and absolute silence. Whereas the feminine practice is about exploring the Shakti aspect, where she dances, sings and surrenders herself fully into worshiping the energy. There is a stronger pull towards the emptiness in the man than in the woman.

This leads us back to the difference between the masculine consciousness and the female energy. The emptiness is more appealing to the man than to the woman. The emptiness scares the woman much more. But speaking of the sexual level, we have a very masculine sexuality in our society, where women have now copied the male sexuality or the part of male sexuality which is focused on how we can get the most sexual pleasure with minimal investment of feelings. Many women are thus drawn to the quick release which leaves her flat: "That took the edge off." So that it no longer feels so frustrating or annoying. The sexual energy is extremely powerful and when we feel it and don't know what to do with it, it can become a source of frustration.

Tantra gives us the tools to direct the energy within and upwards, rather than releasing it. When we direct the energy like this, we feel a deep inner satisfaction when the energy is used to awaken other qualities within ourselves. We call this sexual continence, and it is a source of deep satisfaction.

3. Love

The universe is based on love. Love connects everything. The function of love is to unite. It is like a glue that binds the whole universe together. The entire universe is created from it. It is love that we feel in our hearts and the more we open up to all that love, the more we recognize that we are connected to all that exists.

There are many spiritual paths saying you cannot take anything with you that you have been given in this life, only that which you have given to others. That is the balance we need to find between the material and the spiritual, and we have to understand that by giving, we are getting so much more than by taking.

Especially when we talk about expressing love. To really love, is to love actively, by giving love and manifesting love and acting in the name of love rather than waiting for love, or looking for someone who can love me, so I can love back. The economy of love does not work like that. This is the math of the material life: The more I save, the more I have. But that is not the way love works. The more you give, the more you have.

In tantra we talk about active love. Generally in tantra we speak a lot about yin and yang, the plus and minus, the different energy centres and how they can be out of balance. For most people the heart centre is out of balance at the yin aspect. That means that there is a greater wish to receive love than to give love. We must work with love actively and always give love and translate that love into actions and words, by all the time acting from the present moment and from an impulse in the heart rather than waiting to see: "Will it pay off if I give my love? What will I get in return?" Many people say: "I'll wait until someone loves me, and then he or she can get all my love, but not until then. I choose to give my love to only one person, because I can't cope with loving more than one; that would confuse my mind." Whereas the heart – it is not confused, it just wants to love. The whole idea of loving actively is essential in tantra – in this way we balance our heart.

It also means that in order to have an erotic experience in tantra the heart needs to lead the way. It has to come from a deep wish from the heart to unite with the other person. And a deep wish to give my best to the other one because I love him/her. To love so much that sexuality becomes a natural way of expressing this love and not just a fulfillment of a personal need for pleasure, but rather an expression of "This is the most beautiful way we can unite, right now." "It is the ultimate way I can give you the best of me." When this happens, it becomes so obvious that the sexual experience will change completely, because now it is no longer just two human beings trying to get as much pleasure as possible from each other. It becomes a wish to give the best to each other and to make the other one as happy as they can be.

It is important to be able to both give and receive and it is not enough only to be able to give to the other. You must also be open to receive what you have just given to the other person. When both lovers have learned how to give and how to receive, the magic will happen, and both hearts will be able to synchronize, so they both experience that no one is giving or taking. Everything one of them wants is exactly what the other one wants and together they create magic. At that moment they can share an unspoken experience of both of them doing exactly the right things at the right time. They touch in the right way and in the right places. They change positions at the right time, they make love in a pace that fits both and everything comes together in a higher unity, instead of it being only a sexual encounter during which they both try to get as much pleasure out of it as possible. As it is in the normal situation of with two people who have learned enough about each other to avoid conflict and who have an unspoken agreement to rub against each other's genitals for as long as it works out for them. And who are prepared and willing to replace their partner with a new or better one if it does not work for them any longer.

The tantric relationship is obviously a completely different experience, because the pure sexual experience that only focuses on pleasure is an expression of our modern consumer society. We use each other sexually and as long as we are getting desire and pleasure out of it, it's alright. And once we have "used it up" we must find a new relationship that we can consume. People have gotten used to this throwawaymentality of girl and boyfriends, and it can be a lot of fun and can bring a lot of pleasure. But building a deeper and broader relationship where you can help and support each other in growing – that requires the hearts to be in it a dedication from the heart.

4. Transfiguration

The last cornerstone is transfiguration.

Transfiguration is the ability to see beyond the immediate appearance. It is the ability to see with the soul's eyes rather than the logical eye. It means that when we look at another human being, we see not only their body and personality, but we see the depth of the soul, the spark of the divine that person has within. We can see all the amazing qualities and abilities which are hiding, even if they are at the moment completely undeveloped, and are only small seeds within that person.

If for example I see a beautiful quality in my beloved, that has not been expressed yet, but is only dwelling in its potential form, then just by observing her and that quality it can gradually be awakened. More specifically, you could say that transfiguration is essential for the tantric lovemaking.

Already before the two lovers start their lovemaking they would transfigure themselves and each other. They will see themselves respectively as Shiva, the masculine cosmic consciousness, and Shakti, the female universal energy. In other words, they see the divine universal polarity, both within themselves and the other. We are all divine beings but sometimes we forget that in our daily lives. By initiating lovemaking from this perspective, the strong sexual energy will nurture this perception. So instead of being just man and woman making love, then it becomes god and goddess, Shiva and Shakti, consciousness and energy who, in their ecstatic fusion create the whole universe.

An old saying goes: "Beauty is found in the eyes of the beholder." This beauty, as seen through the eyes of the observer, becomes available through transfiguration.

So tantra is about making a connection between polarity, continence, love and transfiguration, the 4 cornerstones of tantra.

Do you have to understand the philosophy and see the whole perspective to pursue tantra?

You don't have to see the whole perspective to pursue tantra. Tantra begins where we are here and now. Actually no one is able to see the whole perspective when they start. It is all about seeing what we can see, and then get started from there.

For some the motivation can be the desire to have a better sex life. For some it might be that they want to be able to last longer in bed or get better orgasms, or maybe they would like to have a better relationship, intimacy or emotional life. Many people are motivated in the beginning by something that does not work and then there are some that are start from a true spiritual aspiration.

Many spiritual paths are very dry or dull, and do not have the power and energy of the tantric path. Therefore many spiritual seekers are drawn by the tantric way – because it manages to walk the spiritual path without cutting out real life.

Tantra means network, in the sense that everything is connected.

To practice tantra you do not have to be able to see the whole perspective. But you have to have the perspective that there is more between heaven and earth.

Without that openness it will become difficult in the long run. Then it will only be tools to get more out of the life we already have, but without really changing anything or doing anything differently. It is like a bonus, but without the change… And that can be difficult, because when we first start to open that tantric goodie bag, then life will start to change. If you are not prepared for that, then the tantric path will feel like a lot of resistance, it will feel dangerous and way too intense. But if you are prepared for the transformation, then the tantric path is like a spiritual highway, because you can grow very fast with tantra.

Do you need to be spiritual to practice tantra?

You do not need to be spiritual to practice it, but again, tantra is a science about the whole human being and spirituality is a part of being human. It is not a quality that we can cut off, just as we cannot cut off our emotions or our sexuality. You can easily begin practicing tantra without feeling spiritual. But most often you will experience a spiritual opening during the tantric practice, and many people therefore become more spiritual by practicing tantra.

I have had students and met many people who did not have a spiritual opening before they learned about tantra, but just because they started practicing tantra, this opening appeared by itself. There are also some who begin practicing for the sake of healing, and then they slowly open up to the sexual energy, because it is a natural part of being human. Some people have never experienced love, so for them it is quite natural to experience that their heart opens more and more and is able to feel more love.

Some people, who never used their intuition, but always attack problems using logic, will naturally open up for their intuition during the process. And the more you work with your own growth and development, the more you will awaken other areas.

So, no you do not have to be spiritual to practice tantra. But one often becomes more spiritual along the way.

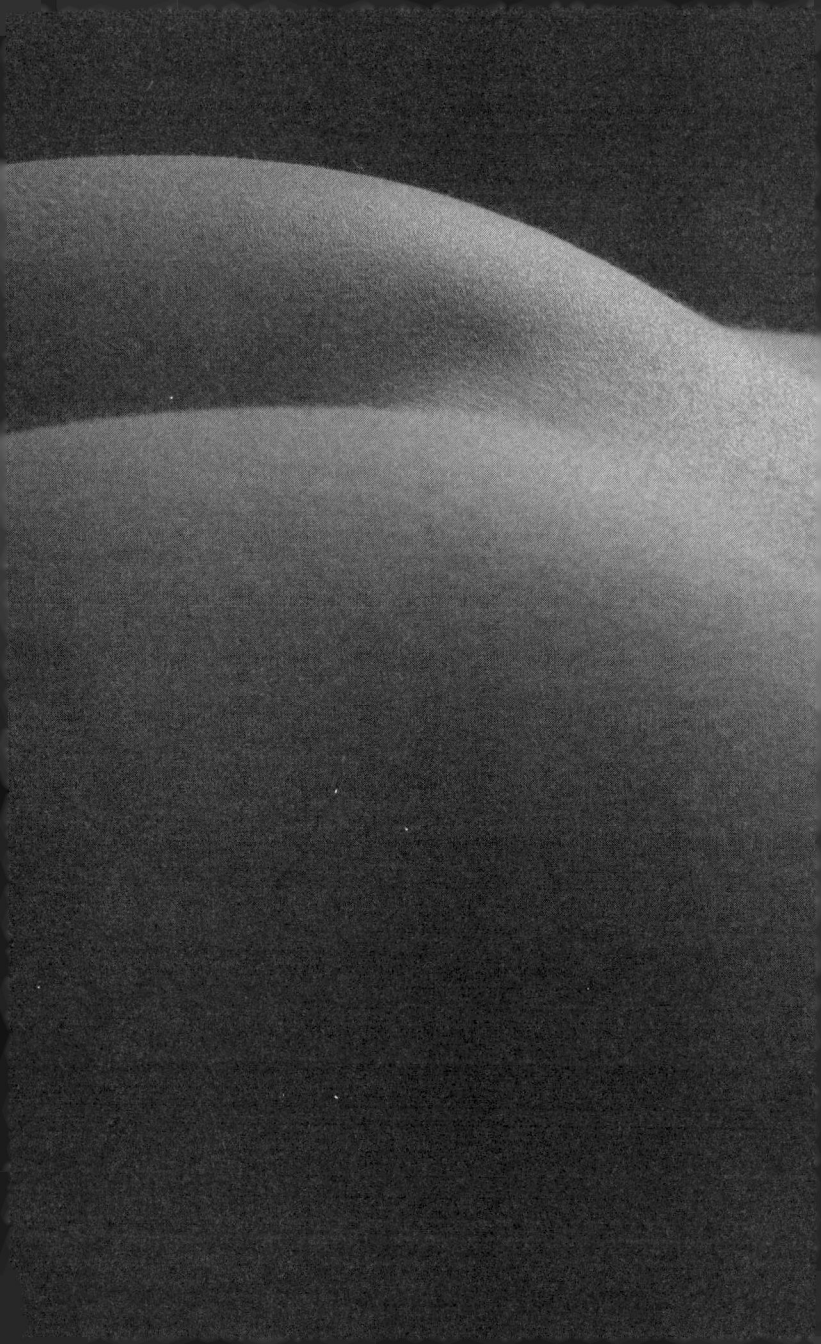

Chapter 3:
Tantra and the whole human being

How does tantra relate to the holistic approach to humanity?

Tantra uses the knowledge of energy from the chakra system to relate to the whole holistic being; and sees the human energy system as divided into seven frequencies, from the lowest frequency to the highest. These energies are not only found in ourselves; but in the whole universe. Thus we have the great universal root chakra and heart chakra etc. As an example, when we awaken, open and balance our root chakra, it will begin to resonate better with the universal root chakra energy. It works like a radio with seven radio stations that we can to tune into. The better we become at tuning in, the better we will be able to listen to that channel.

If we want more vitality, life force, grounding and better stability we have to "play" the root chakra station much more.

Yoga is a very precise tool, if you approach in the right way. Then yoga can become scientific chakra work. The different yoga positions activate the different chakras. If you know which positions activate the different chakras, and if you are able to focus – then you can use yoga as a method to cleanse, empty out, balance, open and awaken every chakra, one by one.

There is just one "but". In order for yoga to become efficient, we have to focus our minds. It's not enough to place our bodies in the right positions and then start thinking about what to post on Facebook when you are done, or what groceries to shop for afterwards. The better we focus our minds on the area that we are working with, the more efficient it will be. This is the an important criteria, and this is also the way resonance works in the broader perceptive. If we wish to awaken more energy in a certain area, then we have to learn to focus long enough on that energy to be able to make a difference. If we only focus on it for two seconds and then think about something else for 10 seconds, then the focus does not have built up enough power. Part of the practice is focusing the mind and staying intensely present in the moment.

Pranayama– breathing techniques is another tool that helps you to focus the energy in a specific area, for instance the root chakra. It can also be an organ that needs more energy. It is possible to speed up the healing process of a poorly functioning liver or an irritated colon or the like. It could also be that you just want to give your lingam more energy, if you want a better erection, a more powerful erection then you can give it more energy with pranayama.

The work of awakening and balancing the chakras requires that you have awareness of them. If you have an understanding of what the different chakras mean and what their impact is, then you can change this impact consciously.

Everything that we do is affected by the awakening or blockage, balance or imbalance we may have in the various chakras. Our basic energy system is the same, but the way it is configured is individual for everyone and thus we are all different. How the chakras work will control our physical wellbeing and our whole physiology, but also our minds – our minds are entirely affected governed by the chakras.

1st chakra: Root chakra Sanskrit: Muladhara

The root chakra governs our life force, vitality, grounding and our ability to have our feet firmly planted on the ground. At the same time it provides us with our instinctive needs; food and sleep, which in return gives us more power and energy to all our processes in life. There has to be a certain amount of awakening in our root chakra for us to be stable in our emotions. If the root chakra is not functioning very well, we will experience that our emotions are very unstable and that our minds drift from one thing to another, and then also our sexuality will lose power. We might feel a lot of lust, but it burns out quite quickly. However, if the root chakra works, it is like putting hardwood on fire. It will burn for hours.

The root chakra is also named Muladhara in Sanskrit, this means the foundation of the root. The root chakra is like the root of a tree and its roots stick into the ground. If they don't go very deep, then the crown will not be able to reach very high either.

Fear is connected to the root chakra. Fear is one of our basic human emotions. It's connected to our instinct. In the root chakra we find our physical as well as emotional survival instinct. When the root chakra is our predominant chakra, we try to protect ourselves from dangerous situations, including the emotionally dangerous ones. By working with the root chakra you will be able to eliminate fear in general. This goes for all kinds of fears – whatever it may be. Many people live their lives in some state of fear.

When the root chakra is fully open and functions well, we are able to get rid of the fear. We will discover a completely different trust in life and that life is not out to get us, and then we can start to enjoy living. To be in existence is also connected to the root chakra.

The root chakra is like a battery. It provides energy to all the processes in our body. And it affects everything that we do.

If it does not function optimally you will not be able to make love for a long time. You will simply become tired after a short while. And if we fall in love, it feels as if we are unable to love more, it seems overwhelming and tiresome to love that much. The emotions are very unstable when the root chakra is not properly awakened. On the other hand, if the root chakra is powerfully awakened, we will fall in love beyond any doubt and be able to stay in love without tiring from the intense feeling.

If the root chakra is lacking strength, there is not much power to draw upon and all the processes run slow and falters.

2nd chakra: The sexual chakra Sanskrit: Svadhisthana

This chakra is governs our sexual energy, but also the way we interact with other people at the social level. As the root chakra was about me and my own survival – the sexual chakra is about survival of the species and of society. It revolves around the group of people that you associate with, it is about fitting in, and the whole idea of fashion stems from this level.

Creativity is also controlled by this chakra. The sexual energy is basically the symbol of creativity and it is the most creative energy of them all. It is also the energy that can create new life. None of the other energies are able to do that. This energy brings life into our lives. It is actually this chakra that plays a role when you have an impulse to create – no matter if it's a project, art or something else you wish to express. This is where you find your creative power.

It is the same energy with which we create children which also brings life and nourishment to for example a painting, that that you want to birth. Whether it is a song, a book, a project or something else we want to bring to life – this is the energy we use. In respect to the root chakra I spoke about having erotic vitality, a good strong life force at the sexual level. At the sexual chakra we talk about the "turn on mechanism". The question is whether the power we have is activated or not. If we have a wellfunctioning sexual chakra, then we will also have a healthy and balanced sexuality with plenty of desire, but without this desire controlling us. If the desire ends up controlling us, then it is because our sexual chakra is off balance. Then you start doing stuff you do not really want to do, because the energy is too powerful and you are not able to control it. Everything from rape to abuse can happen in this situation, but also just plain stupid things that you will regret afterwards. And so you might end up destroying your marriage or getting pregnant by mistake, simply because the desire felt so strong at that particular moment, and you failed to consider the consequences. This is a sign that this chakra is out of balance.

It can also be out of balance in a different way, where you have the desire to do lots of things but end up inhibiting yourself from it. It is the opposite imbalance, where the sexual energy is not allowed to be expressed or only expressed in a very limited way. Maybe you don't behave in an erotic way that often, or that the sexual chakra is blocked so you cannot feel desire.

The sexual chakra has to do with the pleasure of the senses, or pleasure in everything, enjoying what you do or doing the things you enjoy.

When we talked about the root chakra, we spoke about comfort. When focusing on the sexual chakra the focus is on feeling good. Here you want to feel good, cosy and delicious. You do the things you like until you do not like them anymore, at which point you just stop doing them. When your focus is on this chakra, you do not engage into things that are too difficult, even if the reward is really good. What you do has to feel easy or at least comfortable.

3rd chakra: Power chakra Sanskrit: Manipura

The third chakra, named Manipura in Sanskrit, is the power and personality chakra. At the root chakra it was about the theme was one's own survival, and at the sexual chakra it was about the survival of the species. At the personality chakra, the focus is on the survival of the ego, and the impact of the ego on the world. "Watch out, here I come. The focus is on me and what I want". At this chakra we awaken confidence, willpower and the discipline to live your life according to higher principles. It is all about our drive and our ability to manifest our dreams and convert our ideas into reality. If focus remains at the sexual chakra we are able to come up with lots of great ideas, but they will never amount to anything. When the energies in the third chakra are awakened, we will be able to realise our ideas. The third chakra is also connected to our digestion and our inner fire which is capable of metabolizing food. When this chakra works well, we will also have a wellfunctioning digestion, good selfdiscipline and the ability to pursue our own goals.

If this chakra is out of balance, it can manifest in two ways: Either you become very submissive, and then you just do what other people tell you to do, with no regard for your own will. The opposite of that is the tyrant, who tries to manipulate and dominate others, and acts from a very egocentric perspective.

If this chakra is not very awakened, we do not have the power to do much of anything. We can have all the good intentions, a good heart and good ideas, but the power to bring it into the world is missing.

If we define the root chakra as the battery, we can define the third chakra as the engine. However, even with a really good battery – a weak engine will either move very slowly, or not move at all.

4th chakra: Heart chakra Sanskrit: Anahata.

This energy centre is where we experience all the higher human emotions: love, compassion, kindness, altruism and generosity. It holds the wish that things shouldn't only be as I want it, but it should be good for all of us. The well being of others is just as important as my own. I do not want to hurt other people just so that I can get what I want. At the heart chakra level we lift ourselves up above the instinctive, and this is what makes us human. When the heart chakra is well awakened, it is much more open towards other humans. Here we begin to connect with others with the understanding that the others are real living souls just as ourselves, that no matter what colour, conviction, belief or whatever, they are not different from us. We will naturally feel a lot of love for other people, as well as act out of that love and do good for others. We are capable of putting our own needs and egocentric wishes aside in order to help others.

If the heart chakra is not very awakened, we are not able to feel much love. And our emotions are weak. So when we fall in love, the highest expression of that love could be "He/she is kind of cute".

Of course an imbalance of the heart chakra can also make us very focused on the love we want to get. This is where we can become very passive and hesitant in our approach to love and say "Well…. I'm not in love with anyone right now and I have not been for a long time. But if someone comes along and loves me, then I will love that person back". This is a very passive way to approach love. On the other hand, our heart chakra can also be out of balance in such a way that we take advantage of other people's emotions and manipulate them. Maybe even using emotional blackmail such as "If you love me, you do this and that".

5th chakra: Throat chakra Sanskrit: Vishuddha.

The throat chakra relates to our sense of the subtle aspects of life, meaning everything that is not logical and directly perceptible. For instance: When we talk about energies, it requires a certain amount of awakening of the throat chakra to feel phenomena that are not physical. This also goes for feeling energy in the form of vibrations and feeling the more subtle aspects; and being able to understand something which is mysterious and beyond logic.

We use this energy centre for communication; the ability to convert our inner universe into something other people understand. This includes our body language and our subtle communication, but definitely also our verbal communication.

Symbolism is also a subtle way of communication. A plain symbol can communicate a wide range of information. It requires an open throat chakra to be able to understand what a symbol means. Our words are symbols.

The word Vishuddha means clarity, the centre of clarity. The more we activate this chakra, the more we will cleanse all our energies, and the more everything becomes crystal clear and clean, and then we will be able to tell things apart and know what is what. We become able to categorize our experiences, and they will no longer seem like one big blurry mess. This cleansing also takes place in our communication our language becomes clearer. We automatically clean out the extra words that tend to creep into our sentences, like "You know what I mean" or "Ummm" or whatever meaningless words we just add to our sentences.

A person whose throat chakra is not very awakened might feel that communication is difficult, and he or she might have a hard time converting his/her inner world into something that others can understand. Expressing thoughts and feelings may be very difficult, or it might never happen. This person might have a weak and powerless voice, and he/she might find it difficult to understand when people talk about energies.

The yoga I practice always begins with warmup exercises, and the first exercise is a throat chakra exercise. This is simply because then there is a much better chance that the rest of the yoga practice becomes more successful – because you begin by awakening the ability to feel what is beyond the physical. We expand our consciousness beyond the physical and become conscious about the body of energy surrounding our physical body enabling us to feel fine vibrations.

With an open throat chakra we also awaken our intuition more and more. Intuition is an amazing tool once we awaken it and begin to use it, and trust that our intuition is the connection to a deep and underlying truth. It is actually a tool which we can use as a guidance to in life. If we are only guided by our logical sense, we risk missing out on the kind of experiences that our soul needs in order to grow and learn, and then we cannot complete the mission that we are put on this planet to fulfill. It is not necessarily in the best interest of our soul to choose the highest paying job – as our logical sense will often tell us to. Therefore the throat chakra is very important – it helps us connect with the spiritual dimensions of life.

6th chakra: The third eye or mental chakra Sanskrit: Ajna.

This chakra is governs our memory, our intelligence and our ability to focus. The ability to focus is essential, as our mind functions as a kind of tuning device. Let's go back to the mental image of the radio and the seven channels. If the seven chakras are the seven channels, then our mind is what we use to tune in with. When we maintain focus on a phenomenon, an energy, a chakra, then we will attract that energy, and the more we attract that energy, the more it will accumulate in our being.

If we want to work with an energy, it requires that we are capable of focusing long enough on that energy to actually get into resonance with it. If, on the other hand, the mind is completely out of control, jumping back and forth, thinking about anything that comes to mind, then it is not possible to focus long enough to actually build up more of the energy that we want in our lives.

We can call it a kind of mental hygiene. We care a lot about our physical hygiene, and we shower almost every day and make sure that we are clean and nice, and that our belongings and our home are nice, but we don't focus all that much on our mental hygiene. Our mind is filled with so much garbage, mental garbage, things we did not process properly, things we misunderstood. All the things that just go round and round in the mind. Conceptions about the future, or memories about the past – our mind is not present here and now. The mind is always revolving around something, something that has happened, or something that might happen, the past or the future. Even if we feel that we are present in the moment, we relate it to something that we have heard before, or contemplate what it might mean in the future. When we start to get the mind under control, then we will be able to stop the chaotic stream of constant thoughts, and just be present. When that happens, the mind actually begins to function as it should, and to be reflective.

If we have had a powerful awakening of this chakra through intense practice, we will begin to awaken some of the supernatural abilities, such as telepathy, clairvoyance, etc.

7th chakra: Crown chakra Sanskrit: Sahasrara.

The crown centre, the seventh centre, is the crowning glory. It is located at the top of the head and above the top of the head, and it is much more than an energy centre. It is our opening towards the divine and spiritual. Many spiritual traditions talk about this as the channel through which the spirit is channeled into matter. This is where our spirit enters our body. This is something that has been recognised in many traditions, such as the tradition of monks, who shave that part of the head, or others who only keep the hair on that spot. The Jews carry their kippah as a symbol of this being the area of contact with the divine. For many people the crown centre is an area that is very weakly awakened. When it is very little awakened, we do not have a personal experience of the divine.

Through the crown chakra we experience a connection with the divine. It is through this centre that we may experience that our consciousness is much, much greater than we perceive ourselves to be. This is where we can connect with the cosmic consciousness and experience that in reality we are all parts of the same consciousness.

With the awakening of the crown chakra, we begin to experience a direct connection to the divine, and that it is not something far away or something that is separated from us. Nor is it an old grey bearded man in the heavens, that we are not a part of, and who decides over our lives and whom we are trying to please.

The divine is something that we all are a part of, something that is greater than ourselves. The awakening of the crown chakra gives us a new perspective on our own existence, so that we can move away from seeing things from an egocentric perspective. We move from a focus on our own likes and dislikes, and our ideas of what is good for us or not, to a spiritual experience, where every experience we have makes sense. Where both the good and the bad make sense, and where we are able to recognize the lesson within every experience. We can see what our soul needs to experience, and what we need to learn, even in the worst adversity. Whereas before everything was dualistic, we are now able to see that good and bad are just different aspects of the same thing.

The crown centre is, unlike the other energy centres, not dualistic. At the seventh energy centre we are above dualities, there is no yin nor yang. This chakra can be more or less open. It means that we are above the dualistic perception of the world, and we can now begin to see that "the bad" is just as important as "the good".

The more we awaken the crown chakra, the more we will begin to observe ourselves and our own spiritual development wisely. We start to view our life as one long sequence, instead of only seeing the here and now. We can see all the events that we have been through and that they have been essential steps on the journey to where we are now. It gives a clear sign of what kind of lessons will come later in life and the understanding that if I do not learn from this current situation, it will repeat itself. Maybe the lesson will come in a different form, but the essential lesson will be the same. It might be recurring problems in our relationships that will repeat themselves because we need to learn from them. We will also see that once we have gained the wisdom hidden in the lesson, things will change and the problems will not recur.

We can compare life here on earth with a school, a place to learn how to be a human being with all our qualities and challenges. Sometimes we need to take the same class over and over again, while others learn faster, and some people face big challenges in areas that others might find very easy.

From the crown chakra we learn to see the higher perspective, we can observe ourselves without getting hung up on what is good or bad. It is through this awakening of the crown chakra that we begin to feel these really intense spiritual experiences, like for example as Samadhi, or a state of divine ecstasy. Such experiences are life changing. If you get glimpses of how the whole universe is connected and how all of mankind is connected, it will forever change your life. When you have experienced that, there are some things that are impossible to go back to.

Please talk a bit about how the body is viewed from a tantric perspective?

The body is very important and the tantric practice quite often begins with the physical body; a better understanding of the physical body and a better connection to the physical body through the senses. And an understanding that everything is connected, not only through the chakras, but also through our subtle layers of energy.

At the core we have the physical body, surrounded by the energy body, that is a bit larger than the physical body. Then we have the layer that we call the aura or astral body, which is the layer that is made up of our thoughts and emotions – we are actually walking around as twothree meters big thoughtbubbles, that clairvoyants can see as colours. On top of that we have the supramental layer, which is even bigger and much more essential, it is at this level we are perceiving archetypes, and this layer is no longer individual, but universal.

The last layer is "the body of bliss", a very refined layer, that is pure bliss. If happiness has a reason, then bliss has no reason. It is the backdrop of our life, and the one that our mind continuously tries to escape and limits us from seeing; this fully ecstatic bliss that is behind it all. These five layers hide our true essence, our divine Self, in Sanskrit named

Atman. That spark of divinity we all carry within us, that is unalterable, and not individual, but universal.

What guidelines are there in tantra? And what can tantra do for us?

In tantra there are some moral and ethical rules, based upon the concepts that in Sanskrit are called Yama and Niyama, that can guide you when you start your spiritual journey. When you begin your journey, you awaken a lot of energies and then you can use them to make sure that you are moving in the direction for the better. These guidelines are not meant to be dogmatic rules that exclaim: "You may not......", because in the end, tantra says: "Be conscious about the consequences of your actions and then choose freely from that awareness."

This can seem paradoxically for many people who thought that tantra was about being totally free and without taboos, and actually we DO not have taboos in tantra. The guidelines are meant as road signs, and not as roadblocks. They are meant to point out a beneficial direction for all the energy that is being awakened, when you start your spiritual practice.

So, many of the guidelines are not meant to be like for instance the 10 Commandments found in the Bible. The Commandments are like taboos and roadblocks, telling us: "You may not to go that way" and "You may not take this path either". This is the easy way to keep the flock from straying.

Tantra takes the opposite approach: "You can go wherever

you want". There are no taboos, no roadblocks... But there are some signs on the way that you can look at, use for navigation, so that you know whether or not you are on the right track. For instance if you see your actions often hurt other people, it is probably a sign that you are not on the right track because tantra tells us that we are all connected.

The guidelines are:

1. **No violence.** This goes back thousands of years in the tantric tradition; that you should always strive to avoid violence and doing harm to others and yourself. This is of course a very sensible rule, but a very interesting one from a spiritual perspective. Tantra tells us that we should avoid violence in both our thoughts, words and actions. Because everything is connected, even our thoughts of doing harm to others, or negative thoughts about ourselves, are an act of violence. When we do so, we emit a violent field of thoughts. We emit violent energy, and even if we do not act upon it or speak it out loud, we attract violent energy. As long as we have the violence inside of us, we also find violence surrounding us some way or another. We can only move on in our spiritual development when we do away with this. We get rid of it by beginning to to purge ourselves of it, and becoming aware of how much we can hurt ourselves when we think negative thoughts about ourselves and others. At the same time, on a subtle level, we are damaging that other person, because we are projecting negative energy towards him/her. From a spiritual

perspective this will always be something that holds us back. In tantra we are working with the awakening and release of more energy and to allow the energy to flow more freely. Therefore it is natural that we are interested in clearing out all negative trends, both consciously and unconsciously because when we awaken more energy, we pass that energy onto what is already there, this cannot be avoided.

2. To **speak the truth** is one of the important guidelines. It is important to remember, that it is not meant as a command, with punishment for any lies you might tell, but rather about speaking and acting truthfully in regards to what is right to oneself – everything which is true from a spiritual perspective. This also includes a stop to the lies we tell ourselves and complete honesty about where we are right now, and how we can become a better version of ourselves, instead of just doing what you think is comfortable and avoiding what is not. The truth is highly treasured in all spiritual traditions.

3. **You should refrain from stealing.** The desire to own something that belongs to others will not lead you in a good direction. If we see someone have something we would like, for instance money, a car, a girl/boyfriend etc., it will only bring negativity into our lives if we try to take it from him/her. Generally the desire to own other peoples values can lead to serious mental and emotional imbalances. If you steal you are a thief. But

even just wanting something that belongs to another person goes against this principle. Instead we should learn to attract that same thing in our own life. Instead of stealing from others, we can learn to awaken the same qualities in ourselves and when we stay in that resonance long enough, we will begin to attract that situation or those things that we desired to begin with.

4. Not **wasting energy in any way.** To recycle all the energy we have and not only recycle it, but use it for higher purposes. At the sexual level this means that the man should not ejaculate, and that the woman should not ejaculate through explosive orgasms, which drain her energy. That she also learns how to recycle her menstruation within the body, and how she can revert the flow of blood. Instead of a lot of energy spilling out with the blood every month, she teaches her physical body and the energy body how to use this energy for higher purposes. We should learn to control or master our own energy on all levels, not only on the sexual level, instead of losing it for no reason. We call this sexual continence. It can also be about avoiding loss of energy at the physical or material level. Many people have experienced an economic ejaculation; when you suddenly spend money on something that wasn't necessary. But it can also be at other levels, an emotional explosion, instead of working with the emotions at a conscious level, you just explode and then later regret. From a tantric perspective, instead of losing control, you

should consciously work with the emotion and acknowledge every emotion, whether it is powerful, bad or good – it is still energy, and energy can be moved around. No one says it has to stay stuck.

5. To **avoid accumulating things and avoid being possessive.** That you always only possess what is necessary, and avoid cluttering your life with all kinds of stuff you do not need. Material possessions that inhibit and restrict you, keep you locked into a job, a situation, a house, that you can not leave, and which keeps you from doing what is right for you right here and now. Maybe you have a plan for how your life should be, but from a spiritual perspective you have to be willing to give it all up, and move on when you need to move on. It is the complete opposite to the material perspective, where you need to own more and more, and where your bank account needs to grow bigger and bigger, and you need to own larger bigger houses etc. Tantra does not ask you to get rid of everything you own and live an ascetic life, where you just sleep on your yoga mat. Tantra says "Use the things that are necessary, but get rid of the things you do not need, because they will only inhibit and limit you." If we dedicate our life to protect the things we own, then we lose the chance of personal growth. We die while we are still alive.

6. **Purity at all levels.** You have to purify yourself thoroughly inside and outside – a purity both in the

physical appearance and the inner physical world, but also on the mental level. This means cleaning out negative thoughts, a kind of mental hygiene. The energy system of most people is blocked up by chemical and industrial processing of our food, exaggerated consumption of alcohol, tobacco, drugs, heavy metals, toxins in the water, noise pollution, air pollution etc. We need to detox, so the energy can move around freely. But it also means to awaken the senses more intensely, so that the reality becomes more real and intense. I usually recommend to my students that they cleanse tongue, eyes, and nose every day.

7. A **contentment and deep acceptance** of everything being what it is, and letting go of the dissatisfaction with yourself and everyone and everything around you. It is not a passive acceptance like for instance: "I can not do anything about it anyway", but rather a wise, active acceptance and understanding of situations. It is an ability to use every situation to learn something new in life. There is a hidden gift in everything that happens to us, and by understanding that, we can enjoy life without feeling that the world is our enemy. We can also see the joy of what is, what we have, and what has been given us. But it is important to acknowledge that this joy of life and the feeling of satisfaction is something that we find within ourselves, and not a result of outer influences. We should not place any walls between ourselves and happiness.

8. **Fire,** the inner burning passion, motivation and enthusiasm, which constantly drives us forward. We should not sulk and be dissatisfied, but at the same time not just resign and say: "Everything is fine, I just have to sit here and do nothing". Tantra says: "Act, be active, and awaken even more of this inner burning fire, that makes you take action, here and now, if you know this action is the right thing to do. Feel it in your heart and do it. Do not wait for the right moment to say and do things, thinking that there is a better moment than now". We must move on, we need to act and at the same time be satisfied. Not satisfied with the way things are, but a deep feeling of satisfaction with everything we do. Instead of just doing what you love, then love what you do, put your whole soul into it, and make it come alive.

9. To **study** and strive to learn more about who you are and about the world, and continue growing, understanding and expanding your horizon, especially from a spiritual perspective, and always aiming to reach a deeper understanding of the question: "Who am I"? With this I do not mean to just accumulate information, but to build a greater understanding of ourselves and recognition of our true nature. To study those who have gained such a deep recognition of their higher Self for instance through books, lectures, or by directly seeking counseling from a spiritual guide.

10. **Acknowledge** that we are all part of the divine at all times. That it is not me against the world, but that we

are a part of everything that exists. That everything happens for a reason. That every situation that we experience carries a lesson from which our soul can learn. If you are stuck in your ego, then every situation will be perceived as either good or bad. If you have a bad experience then you will try to blame others, and then you lose the chance to learn the lesson – this spiritual principle is an attitude that will change the inner perspective. In the western world we have a powerful egodriven culture, therefore the act of just surrendering can feel like a defeat. In war or in any other game we can give up and surrender to the greater power by giving the others the victory. But tantra transforms this "surrendering" from being just the last resort to a constant practice. The victory is gained by freely and constantly giving up our limited ideas of who we are, and by that I mean our name, our job, our problems and so on. Thereby we create the space to feel our true nature, and the spark of eternity that we all carry within us.

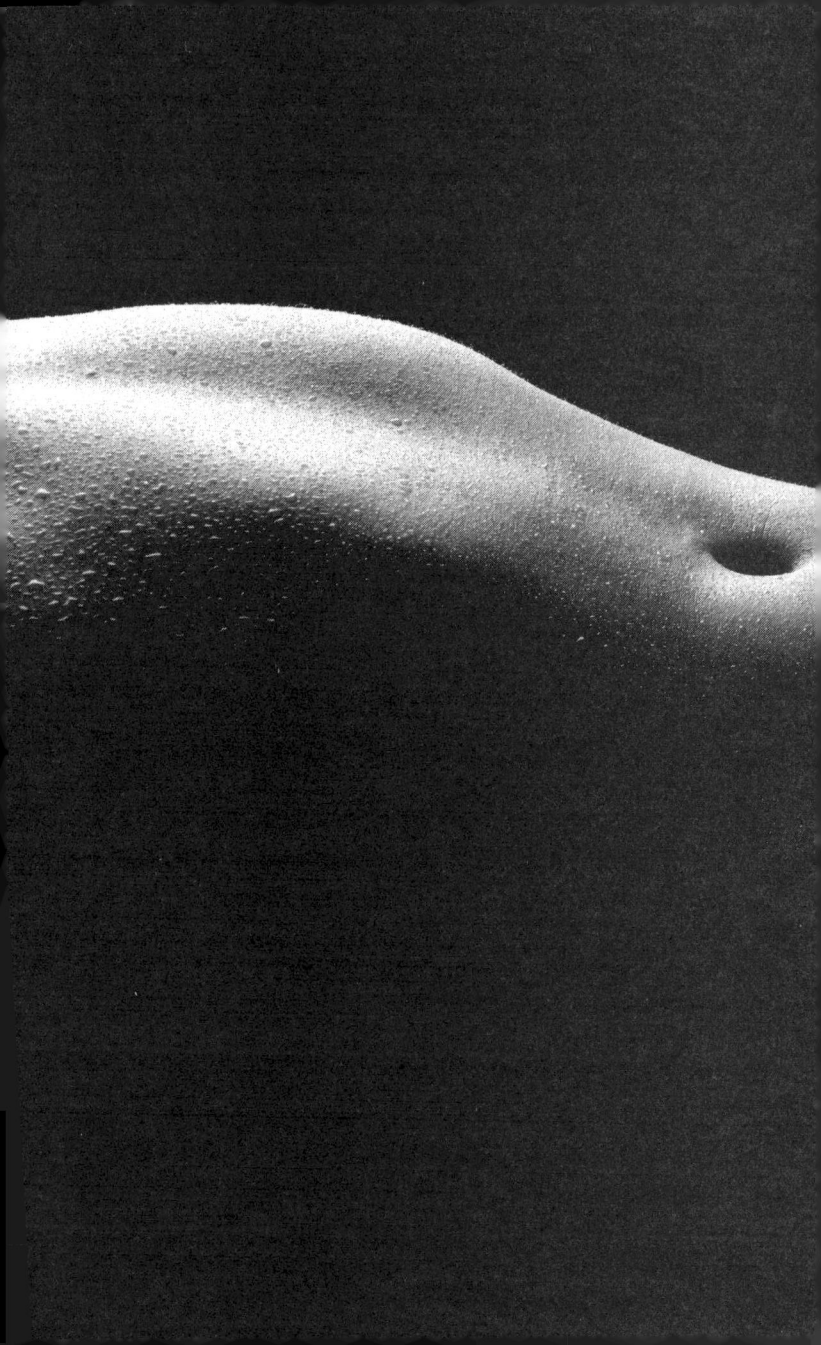

Chapter 4:
The tools of tantra

We have talked about the tools in tantra, what can you say about that?

The tools are:

1. To quiet the mind.

Part of the tantric practice consists of quieting the mind, simply meditation and concentration exercises to turn off the mind, to actually be able to listen to what the right choices are.

The soul is constantly giving us directions, issuing orders about the right actions in any given situation in order to gain the insights that we here to learn. But the mind always yells louder than the soul if we allow it. Thoughts then loop around in our head, and every time we are faced with a decision, the mind does what it is here for. It analyses, weighs the pros and cons, and begins to add the two sides up against each other. The mind is not created for decision making.

Decisions are made with the heart. We know immediately what decision to make, when we are placed in certain situations, but immediately the mind starts presenting the pros and cons. We are raised not to make decisions without a good reason, and that this reason has to make sense, it has to be logical. An important part of the tantric practice is to get so much control of your mind that you can quiet the mind and listen to the voice of your heart. We just need to know that the voice of the heart is not loud. It has a very fine and sweet voice, that we are only able to hear when the mind is quiet.

The process of surrendering yourself to listen to that voice, even if you do not always agree with it, makes life much more beautiful, but people often don't know that.

Some people venture into personal growth and discover that they have a voice, a voice from the heart, and then they begin the process of learning how to listen to that voice. But there are also many people who are unaware of this choice they have. It doesn't matter where you are in life, whether you are preoccupied with a professional career or spiritual practice or if you have your focus on your family life or whatever it may be… Tantra is helping you to see where you are at right now. It helps you to see all your good qualities, all your obstacles and challenges, and also all the aspects you do not wish to face in your daily life.

Tantra offers you all the tools you need to openly and honestly analyse yourself and say: "How can I get even closer to the perfect version of myself"? At the same time it also gives you the tools you need to make the desired changes. That means the ability to change what you have discovered about yourself, for example: "Maybe I should become better at opening up my heart", "Maybe I need more confidence", or "Maybe I need a more balanced approach towards my own sexuality" or whatever it might be that you have to acknowledged openly and honestly.

Many believe that the phrase: "Free your mind" is very tantric, but it is not. "Free your heart, free your soul" is much more tantric, also, rather than saying "Free your mind", we would say "Discipline your mind". Because the two; our mind and our heart, often work against each other. The mind is just a tool we can use whenever we need to use logical thinking to figure something out. Besides that, it should keep quiet and remain still, and thereby allow us to hear the voice of our heart.

2. Pleasure

Pleasure is a tool used in tantra. Therefore there are tantric techniques to awaken more pleasure. But if we lose focus on why we are doing this, then we are missing the whole point. Pleasure is used as a tool to gain a higher state of consciousness. Pleasure is used to awaken all aspects of ourselves; we have been given the power of creation and all we need to do is to give it back on a spiritual level. When we do this, pleasure becomes a super fantastic and super powerful tool. If we lose sight of this goal and make pleasure the only goal, then it makes no sense.

This might be a lot of fun. But it would be like having a car just for driving it around, but having nowhere to go. Just for the fun of driving around, but never getting anywhere, that would be a pity. Unfortunately, many people think that this is what tantra is all about, but when the essence is removed it can no longer be called tantra, but maybe pleasure therapy instead.

3. The tantric setting

When we speak of tantric massage, it is not so much about the massage techniques as it is about the tantric setting. It is about having the right tantric attitude and the right understanding of the tantric principles – of why we are working with sexual energy? Why are we working with pleasure? Why are we working with polarities? The attraction between the masculine and feminine? And where are we going with all this? Understanding the energy, how it flows and how we can help open it up. First and foremost all this needs to be in place, and then we can choose whatever massage technique we want.

If you were to film a tantric massage, and give the video to a professional masseur, with the request for him to copy the massage, it would not become a tantric massage, because he will not gain the understanding of what is actually taking place by simply copying the technique. It is essential to understand and the reason why tantric massages can differ so much.

What one guest needs can be very different from what another guest needs. The massages can vary from a very powerful and dynamic touch to an extremely soft touch, where you do not even touch the physical body, but only work at the energy layer around the body. It can vary this much and also be all of this in one single experience encompassing all these different phases. It can be one long sequence, an embrace, while working in complete awareness, with the conscious touch running through everything that takes place.

The tantric massage seeks to unite the two; to help both the receiver and the giver go beyond their own egos and experience a close human connection. The tantric experience, whether it is in the form of a massage or lovemaking, aims towards union, because when we learn how to unite with another person, then we have already taken a very important step in becoming more human.

The tantra massage helps the guests unite with themselves. The movements and energy of the masseur helps us feel ourselves and return to our true nature, thereby radiating what we truly are.

4. The tantric attitude

Everything can be a tantric technique, if you have a tantric attitude. At the tantra course I am teaching, I use all kinds of theories and exercises from many different paths and systems. Tantra means network, the connectedness between everything, so just because a certain technique was invented by another spiritual path or system, it does not exclude it from being used in tantra.

But in order to call something a tantric massage, there has to be a tantric frame and within that frame you can use all kinds of techniques. Many people believe that tantric massage is a technique, but it isn't. Tantric massage is an attitude, and it can entail all kinds of touch.

One tantric attitude you can practice in everything you do, is the combination of relaxation and attention. Only when we are fundamentally relaxed are we able to expand our awareness and our consciousness. As soon as our attention is not based on relaxation, it will be limited. When we need to focus on something and tell ourselves to: "Buckle up"! we have already made a frame for ourselves with clenched teeth and squinted eyes. This kind of concentration will always be limited. At some point you will not be able to tense up anymore.

On the other hand, when attention is based upon deep relaxation it is unlimited. Many people relate focus to tension, and relaxation to lack of consciousness. "If I am going to relax, then I need to sit in front of the TV, without thinking of anything, and just space out, while something is flickering in front of my eyes". But that is not true relaxation. Maybe we feel that we are relaxed, but in reality a lot of processing is going on in the background.

We are only truly relaxed when we relax as a conscious action. When we just relax without awareness, then our bodies are actually tense in many places. All these small constant tensions in our body have to be let go of in a conscious way. The body does not relax by doing nothing. We think it does, but it doesn't.

Therefore the tantric practice begins with a lot of relaxation, and not just on the yoga mat, but by bringing that relaxation with us into our daily life, and by learning how to be effortlessly relaxed in every situation. Then we will realise all the many situations in where we are much more tense than we need be.

Once you learn how to relax, you will be able to handle much more. Then we can actually find ourselves in situations that we expected would be very stressful, without feeling the least bit stressed. Instead we find ourselves to be resourceful and able to deal with it without freaking out.

The combination of relaxation and attention becomes a tantric practice in everything we do, where we constantly realise how we relax the most by increasing our attention more and more.

5. The senses

In tantra we use our senses extensively, because the senses are like portals to the present moment, and our sensory experiences can only take place in the present. We are so used to being separated from the present moment, because our mind is in control. If we really would analyse our thoughts, we would realise that many of them are dwell in the past. We think about what happened and what could have been done differently. We may even try to make it seem better than it was.

And when we don't think about the past, we think about the future. Thoughts about what the future might bring, or worries about what is ahead cross our minds. Generally speaking the mind is everywhere except in this moment. Thus we are not fully present in our heart, and therefore we are not able to fully love here and now. We are focusing on our expectations of what might happen with this love. Or maybe we are stuck in an old idea of what will happen if we allow ourself to love someone. The point is that when we let the mind take control, then we are not present in the moment. This is where our senses work so beautifully, because they help us come back to the present.

We cannot feel what we felt yesterday, our skin cannot feel tomorrow's touch, we cannot smell or taste the sensations of tomorrow. The senses only work in the present, so the more we focus on our sensory experiences, the more we are present in the moment. As mentioned before, our senses become a portal to the present moment. Once we have learned that, we are able to stay present in the moment regardless of what we are doing, without the need to fully submerge into our senses every time. In tantra we use this as a tool in the practice of staying in the present.

Therefore tantra has tantric rituals to awaken and enter the five senses one by one. Usually it is done in the same order as the first five chakras; the sense of smell, the sense of taste, the sense of sight, the sense of touch and the sense of hearing. The senses are awakened one by one as we give each sense full attention, and try to ignore the others. During such rituals one becomes aware of how much intensity you can find in just one sense. For instance, when you fully taste something, and instead of just passing it through your mouth, you focus completely on the taste and the experience. Or when you feel the touch of a hand on your skin, and surrender yourself fully to this sensation: "Where am I being touched? What is it doing to me? How does it make me feel inside? What does it awaken in me? Would I be able to recognise this hand tomorrow – just through the touch?? Without seeing it, would I recognise the feeling of this hand"? Such intense presence brings us deeply into the moment, and then we are in contact with ourselves, in contact with our soul and then we have the chance to see what is real, and not just projections from the past and the future. We live with a filter, constantly colored by past experiences and expectations of the future.

During a tantric massage it is possible to open up to the sense of touch, and to experience the intensity of the touch. You are given the opportunity to feel your body, in ways and places, that you might never have been touched at, or given attention to before. During a tantric massage you are also asked to be conscious of the touch, to be present with the touch, and not allow the mind to take over and slip away into thoughts. You are asked to follow the touch of the hand, pay attention to what is happening in the very moment and how it makes you feel, whether it be a very firm and powerful touch or one as light as a feather. You are invited to really feel what it does to you and to dive deep inside your own experience of your senses.

In all love making, our five senses are in play, but in the tantric love making we strive to enhance the sensory experience so much that everything becomes connected at a higher level. This means that we smell each other, we look at each other, we taste each other, and we feel each other. We listen to the sounds – not just the music that we have selected – but also the sounds our bodies are making, when they are together, the spontaneous sounds of pleasure we make when me make love, and our breathing. All these sensations merge into a higher awareness, that can keep you present in the moment, and keep you from mentally drifting away into thoughts of other things, or fantasies about someone else. All experiences that bring us away from the present constrict our consciousness. All present experiences, intense experiences we feel in the present moment, will expand our consciousness.

The more experiences like this that we have, the more energy? we are able to contain as our consciousness expands. We begin to experience all kinds of delicate nuances in our senses which we have not experienced before. And we experience the ability to focus on the five senses all together, instead of for example just being very occupied with the visual and not listening, or very occupied by the sense of touch and forgetting to taste and see.

It is truly a tantric practice to awaken the five senses. The more you do this with full awareness, and one sense at a time, the more aware of the big picture you become, and the better you become at realising it when you drift away from the present moment. If you experience that you have moved onto a fantasy, it is better to open your eyes and instead enjoy the reality that is here and now.

Men are often more visual than women. That means that men tend to have their eyes open most of the time, because it arouses them to see a beautiful, naked and sexually awakened woman. It is very stimulating for him, but it keeps him from sensing everything else around him as fully. Women are the opposite. They have a tendency to close their eyes and disappear into thoughts and fantasies. A good practice might be for the man to close his eyes more, and instead feel more, and for the woman to keep her eyes open and remain in the present moment. But most importantly, we must sense what we are doing, what we can improve, and how we can awaken more of ourselves?

6. The analysis
Where do you find guidance if you wish to know more about tantra? Where do you go to learn more? Do you need to go to India or can it be found in the West?

It can be found in the West as well, but amidst challenging conditions, because many people have a difficult time accepting advice and guidance from another person. But still it is essential to find a person, who can guide you on the part of the journey you have not yet walked yourself. A person who is more evolved than yourself in the areas you seek to evolve. There are very few examples of enlightened tantric masters, but they can be found. It does not have to be in the form of a relationship, in which you spend a lot of time with this person, but it can be more like tuning into the field he or she creates from the personal spiritual growth. It's like we tune into the teachings, or the spirit, in which tantra is taught, in order to have a sincere system to follow. As I said earlier, you can find many people who use tantric techniques side by side with all kinds of selfdevelopment techniques, some of them homemade, but that is not tantra. It would be a shame to go too far in the wrong direction, because of the lack of navigation. It is a waste of time to explore a direction path that later turns out to be wrong, and which does not bring us closer to true spiritual growth.

How does the analytical practice work in tantra?

In regards to the chakras you gain both a theoretical understanding, and a very practical individual understanding of your own chakra system. You spend an extensive amount of time learning what it means to you on both the physical, psychological and mental level. You learn how the chakras work when they work, and when they don't.

We actually have some questionnaires that deal with some of the issues; like your sleep pattern for example. For a period, try to notice how many hours you sleep at night, from what hour to what hour, and what time you go to bed. Maybe also take some notes about the quality of sleep. Do you wake up many times at night? Do you feel well rested in the morning? Simply shedding some light on the sleep issue. Casting light of consciousness on different areas of life that you normally don't look at. Like your eating habits: What do you eat? How much do you eat? Are you often hungry during the day? Do you eat, because you have to eat? All kinds of different aspects of the physical life – write it down and then practice on the root chakra, because this chakra is very connected to sleep and food, and then take note of the difference afterwards.

Then you have a starting point. You know that you sleep this much per night, and eat this and this, and that you feel that you have this amount of energy. An example: "I feel drained of energy a couple of hours every afternoon, and then I regain energy for a while, and a couple of hours before going to bed, I feel really tired", or however it might be in your case. Then you practice intensely on the root chakra for a month or two, and check again. Has anything changed? Is it better now? This could be your first practice. Or it can be at the sexual level, and some of the questions here might be:

How often do you make love? How long does it last? Do you have many sexual fantasies? How important is sexuality to you? Simply analyse yourself in this area.

Most people experience great change on the various levels after ½ 1 year of practice, which helps them recognise the value of their practice. Of course yoga, meditation practice and breathing exercises can make anyone feel good, because it feels nice. But it all really begins to make sense when we experience long lasting changes in our lives.

The tantric techniques can provide us with some very obvious and life changing effects.

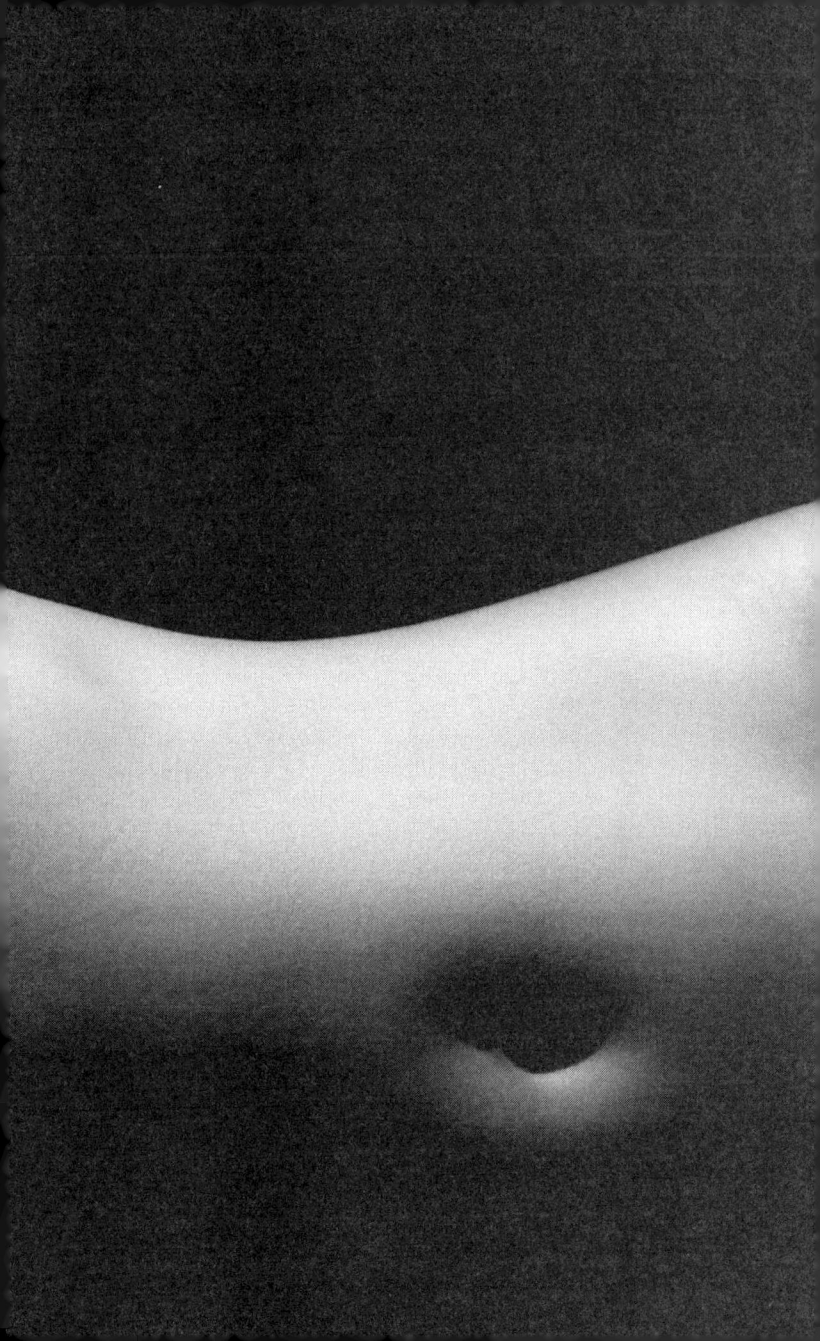

Chapter 5: Tantra on the individual plane

Tantra, what does it mean to me?

"Tantra begins where you are" is a tantric saying. I teach a tantra course, which welcomes people exactly where they are. It is based upon explaining the human system of the seven chakras and the five energy bodies, as we talked about earlier. It explains that: "This is how we are all created, but we are all different, we all have different nuances, different levels of awakening, balances and imbalances". "Those of you who have just begun your journey, start with the discovery of how you are put together. How is your energy system? And how awakened, in or out of balance, are your chakras"? "Openly and honestly analyse yourself from the holistic perspective".

Realise that you are already completely perfect as you are, and that there is a reason why you are the way you are, and that you can awaken an even better version of yourself.

Precisely those sides of ourselves we like the least or turn a blind eye towards are the ones that can make a huge difference in our lives with just a minimal amount of effort.

This is where tantra begins! By recognising where I am right now in my evolution, in my own process, and how to move on from there. Tantra provides all the tools you need in order to analyse yourself completely, openly and honestly. The seven chakras give you an amazing insight to your qualities, as well as your challenges. At the same time tantra provides the tools to do something about it, to work directly on the specific energies. When you discover a side of yourself that you would like to change, you will find the exact methods and techniques to work with the areas that you have become aware of, and then begin to change the energy in these areas. It is not a therapeutic process in which you analyse, or change your patterns of thought, or adapt methods to learn how to live with these flaws. Instead you look at the energy, and then you purify the energy at that level, and thereby you will experience a change in behaviour and thought patterns. This is where it begins at the individual level.

When talking about tantra, some people think that it is something you do with someone, and that you need to have a partner. But it is not like that at all. Well, yes it is something you can do with a partner, but it begins right where you are, right now. When working with the tantric energy in a couple or in the tantric lovemaking, for instance there is a tremendous amount of energy being exchanged, and if you are not yet aware of your own energy, then it is impossible to navigate in that exchange with another person, who does not know their own energy either. Therefore tantric practice begins by getting to know yourself and your own energy. Then later you can benefit from merging your own energy with someone else's. If you would begin by learning tantric love making together, then the techniques and methods can be so affected by your habits and old patterns, that it would be incomprehensible what is your energy and what is the others one's energy during the love making.

If you are in a relationship, tantra suggests you to completely reprogram the way you interact with each other sexually, intimately, emotionally and communicatively. Then afterwards you can begin to experience much higher levels of love making. I mean, we can talk about the man and the woman fusing together at all levels and becoming the cosmic masculine and universal feminine. But if he lies there thinking: "I hope I can keep the erection up long enough and I hope she will do this and that, because I really like that", and she is thinking: "I hope I look good in this position" and wondering if she remembered to do the dishes, and is hoping that he is done soon, because it just feels like he is masturbating inside of her… If that is the case, then there is no fusion of Shiva and Shakti. This kind of situation that we see in this example would require a great deal of individual work for the two lovers.

There are different approaches to Tantra. One says: "You have to work with yourself and your own practice for 20 years, and then finally you can be initiated in sacred sexuality". Another approach says: "Just have sex with as many as possible, as often as possible, and get all the experience you can". It would almost be like running away from the whole experience, if you lock yourself away for 20 years and only practice with yourself until you have reached perfection on all levels. But on the other hand, it does not make sense to just throw yourself into all kinds of experiences with no understanding of what is going on. I believe that instead it should be a balance of practicing with ourselves and gaining experiences with others in order to achieve a greater understanding of what is happening, so that we continuously validate our practice.

Some people come across tantra in the search of a better sex life, and others because of actual problems they would like to heal. It can be physical problems, or mental traumas they would like to let go of, or something else that is holding them back. Some feel just fine, but they are on a quest to experience more at the sexual level, as well as other levels, while others just want to get to know themselves better.

Tantra makes a lot of sense, especially for women when they hear that sex can be much more than just sex as they know it. But a lot of men are also joining this search for something more. The Danish society and Danes in general have an open approach to sexuality, and therefore many people come to the tantric massage with an intention or search in the area of sexuality, for instance:

1. There must be something better.
2. I want to do it better.
3. Or I want to get rid of my problems.

Once they experience that tantra only works through practice and not by merely reading about it, many people open up and ask: "Can tantra do more than this? Can it do more in my life"? And yes, it can, because tantra does not only look at the whole human being, but the whole universe.

Tantra has this fascinating perspective of life or view of the human being, that we humans are a holographic copy of the entire universe – we are actually small universes copied from the big universe. This means that everything I encounter within myself, is something that I can also encounter outside myself at the universal level. At the same time, everything that I can encounter outside is also something to be found inside myself. There is nothing inside of me that I cannot find in the outside world and the other way around. If I want to know and understand the universe, I can look inside myself, and all the answers will be there. Then it becomes a fascinating energy work where we begin to recognise that it is actually not our own energy that we are working with. What we are working on is our energy system and when it is in balance, we are able to open up and thereby allow the universal energy to run freely through us.

When speaking of love, we then don't just talk about "my love". We finally understand that it is not as if I have x amount of love available that I can distribute to a certain amount of people. Love is infinite. There is an abundance of universal love. It is an inexhaustible source, that we are all able to connect to, and it's all about how much we can open our heart chakra and let the energy flow through. The more we do this, the more we also resonate with the universal love. Then it is no longer individual love, which we choose to give to one person and not to another, based upon whether or not we feel that he or she deserves our love. Love becomes more universal, and the more we open up, the more love we feel towards all beings and this is a very fascinating journey. It is not only love that works like this. This is true on all levels.

About the tantric massage.
So tantra is not only about pleasure or satisfaction, but a meeting with the true Self, and that also means that you are not always happy and blissful in massages or lovemaking. Is it not a big misunderstanding that you will always feel happy and joyful in a tantric meeting?

All feelings, both good and bad, are present and increase a thousand times in the tantric meeting, but a lot of those who call themselves tantric masseurs think it is about giving the guest more pleasure. Pleasure is not a goal in tantra. Pleasure is a tool. If you miss that point, you might help people to a better sex life, but you miss the whole point of tantra.

In the tantric perspective we have to take our own life in our own hands. We, as tantra masseurs, are not here to fix people, but to show them qualities in themselves that they are not yet aware of, and therefore we give them the tools to get there. Tantra massage is not something you receive as "a fix", or because you are addicted to it, or because it is the only way to experience this. It is more like a developmental journey, with a "tourguide" on your inner journey, someone who shows you around: "Look at this and look at that. See what you are capable of". "Wow this is fantastic! How do I get there myself?" "Well, yes listen now, you have to do so and so…". And then the actual journey begins. It begins with a leap into yourself, and the "tourguide" is just showing you points of interest. In tantra we are not looking for the occasional tourist, but rather someone choosing to be at home with themselves wherever that may be.

Even if you only come for massage once, a seed has already been planted. The massage is not only about giving a pleasurable experience, but about being fully present in the moment?

Yes, exactly. It is always about this moment and giving everything fully to the present moment.

People come with all kinds of motivations. Some haven't even really understood what it is when they come here for the first time. Some are surprised that it turns out to be something completely different than what they expected. But many of them are positively surprised, because this is something that can change their life. That they are actually able to feel something. To feel energy in a completely different way than they are used to.

What kind of preconceptions do people have?

It differs. Some think it is a sexual experience, and that they are going to experience sexual pleasure. Some think it is only about healing. This is typically people who have problems of some kind or another. It can be a woman with tension or pain in her abdomen, or a man with erectile dysfunction or premature ejaculation. Or a woman who has had many bad experiences with men, and therefore needs to regain the feeling of trust and safety. Many different kinds of people, motivated by many different kinds of problems. Then they realise that tantra massage can help them, not only with that specific problem… but that it can also awaken completely new qualities in themselves that they have been unable to see until now, because they have been limited by the problem or situation they were in.

People who come to the massage with an erotic motivation are often surprised to experience how much love they feel in the situation. Some almost feel anxious because of all the love they feel. They feel surprised that they can actually feel closer to the masseur, than they have ever felt before with another person.

Even though it is not sexual, the experience might feel more intimate than anything they have done before, even with their spouse for the past 20 years. Some find this very fascinating, others are deeply frightened. "Then what? Am I in love with my tantra masseur? That's not good". But in reality, it's not about the feelings you awaken towards each other in the massage, but the ability to open up your heart and to love deeply and sincerely. This is an ability you can bring home into your everyday life, and use in all your relationships and with the people you meet. You can become a more loving person. You can become someone who expresses love and acts out of love. Not many people expect this when they come, and it is not something that we can write on our webpage, because it could be greatly misunderstood. The idea of going to a place to learn about love… it's to strange… people feel that this is something they should do with their beloved, at home. Tantra massage can be many things that people don't expect beforehand but feel moved by. .

Can you clarify how you use the knowledge about energy in the massage?

In the Tantra Temple we have all worked intensely with

our own energy through tantric yoga exercises, meditations, breathing techniques etc. When you have spent thousands of hours on the yoga mat and worked specifically with one exercise in a certain position that awakens a certain energy… Once you have done it extensively, you are able to awaken that energy simply with your willpower, because you have already been there so many times that it becomes a natural state.

During the massage, the masseur is therefore able to open up the various chakras and guide you with the help of energy and without using words.

When speaking of energy, we speak about working with resonance. Resonance is when two somewhat similar energies affect each other and start resonating and unifying more and more. If one is powerful the other one will follow. This phenomena is known in all areas of life. When things vibrate on the same wavelength, they will affect each other. The classic example of this is that when two violins are placed on a table and you strike a string on one of them, then the same string on the other violin will begin vibrating, without even being touched. This happens on the energy level all the time. For example, we all know that when someone is in a good mood, it will impact you, and the same is true if someone brings a bad mood. Of course this only happens if we resonate with that energy.

If we are generally pissed off and cross, it doesn't change just because someone shows up in a good mood, because we just don't resonate with the good mood in that moment. There is simply no opening for the good mood. There is not even a spark of good mood behind the surface that can be awakened. On the other hand, if you are generally in a good mood, you are not affected by someone's bad mood, because you do not resonate with their energy in that moment.

When we speak about connecting sexuality and love, connecting the yoni [the vagina] with the heart, or connecting the sexual energy centre with the heart centre, it primarily means that I, the masseur, am doing that myself. It means that if I tell her: "Now you have to bring your sexual energy up into your heart, so try to breathe in a certain way or focus like this", then I am also myself simultaneously moving the energy in that way. If I awaken enough energy in my heart chakra, it resonates with her heart chakra and it becomes much easier for her to feel her heart. However, if I stay in my sexual energy centre and just tell her: "Now you need to bring the energy up into your heart, and you have to do this and this in this way", then the success would depend on whether she is already able to do it or not, because there is no help from my energy.

It will often have the completely opposite effect if I as masseur stay in the sexual energy centre and, without sincerity and without really being in the heart myself, say: "Now we need to move the energy up into your heart". It would not feel genuine to her. She would need to be very skilled in order to bring the energy up into her heart centre without the help of resonance with my energy. That is a very classical example of how we are able to help people through the work of resonance, and due to our many years of practice.

For thousands of years tantra has been passed on through initiation. The initiated ones pass the initiation on to others, who will then be initiated. This actually means that because of the work with our own energies, we are able to give other people experiences and transformation they could never have achieved alone or with a masseur who has not yet reached that level. This is a very practical way in which we are able to give people profound experiences with their own energy system and help them become aware of their energy.

It is evident that there has to be some form of resonance. There has to be a small opening of the heart chakra before we can help create a bigger one, and there has to be a small opening of the crown chakra for the massage to become a spiritual experience.

Many people are surprised to feel how much love an experience like this can hold and to realise just how much love they can feel themselves. And this is just one example of what they are able to experience. "Yes, you can feel this much love all the time, if you want to. Right now it is just possible, because we create a space where that frequency is dominant." And experiences like this is why the massage can feel so overwhelming, because we are not used to allowing love to dominate our lives.

We are used to feeling it a little bit, but then we allow other things to take control and love slips into the background.

If you create the right space, a room with the right tantric frame and attitude to get the person to relax, and then make the person feel safe while gradually making the massage more and more sensual. When you awaken more erotic energy, and move it up into the heart, then the energy will be so powerful that many feel an unsurpassed opening of their hearts. But again, it is not just about touching the right places, even if that is very helpful the tantric massage is a guided experience made possible by the energy of the masseur.

The tantric massage makes it possible to show the tantric world and show the tantric perspective of intimacy and sensuality without making love to people. The energy and the resonance is being passed on. A lot of men experience themselves in a completely new way, when they are being nurtured by the energy and warm sensual femininity of a female masseuse for two hours or more.

For those who have had problems with premature ejaculation, this is a powerful experience, because they are so used to the experience being over almost as soon as the clothes have come off. They are not used to having the time to experience deep intimate connection or feeling able to be present for their partner. During the massage there is no expectation of him to perform. This enables him to feel his manhood better and gain more control of his energy, to the point where he might even be able to be sexually aroused and maintain his erection for hours, as opposed to minutes. This is profoundly lifeaffirming for a man, and can help his personal growth tremendously.

Exactly the same goes for women who receive a massage. She has an experience with a man who is fully present with her, takes care of her, holds her and helps her feel herself, and who is not in a hurry with anything, or needs to get somewhere specific. This is also quite an amazing experience for many women; both the experience of what it is like to be close with a man, who is in perfect control of his sexual energy, but also an indication of what it would be like to make love in that way. Not that the man makes love to her, but by him showing her ways of being touched that she is not used to, or by being together with a different focus than what she is used to. This can help women become more aware of what they like. Many women experience problems with their sexuality. If the man doesn't know what she likes, she tends to compromise her own desires and instead agree to what he likes. Even if she wants something to stop, it can be difficult for her to express what she would like instead. Her intuition might tell her that sex can be much more than just regular sex. But she cannot explain or express it, because she hasn't experienced it yet.

A tantric massage can show her how it might also feel. "Now I understand why I always had this feeling that something was wrong, even if we did what we were supposed to. Even if I had orgasms, there was always the feeling that something was missing".

For most people there is a great deal of focus on the orgasm. What is the tantric perspective on this?

The orgasm is a fantastic state of being, which brings us beyond our own ego and our own limitations. The problem is that many people never experience how good or how many orgasms they can actually have. Most men are locked in the belief that orgasm and ejaculation are the same thing, but they are not. The man can learn how to have a lot of orgasms without ejaculation, and thus how to become multiorgasmic, just as a lot of women are. It just requires some practice on his part. The woman can learn how to have many different kinds of orgasms and not just quick explosive orgasms from the clitoris.

When wanting to learn how to become multiorgasmic, a lot of men do what I did in the beginning: Instead of focusing on getting an ejaculation, they start to focus on not having an ejaculation. That is not the right way either, that is just avoidance. Instead of focusing on the ejaculation, you have to focus on your ability to become a multiorgasmic man. That means to stay focused on having an orgasm without ejaculation. It is a bit like the tightrope walker, he does not focus on NOT falling down. He remains focused on keeping his balance. Even a tantric master who has been sexually continent for 25 years could get an ejaculation quickly if he wanted to, or if he would let go of his awareness. Exactly like the perfect tightrope walker – he will fall in a split second if he is not aware. But he has practiced and perfected his awareness to the point where he never loses his balance.

This is also true for the tantric man. Even if he has trained, and is capable of coming very close to, but not having, ejaculation, it does not free him up to think about something else or mean that he cannot ejaculate. He is just so intensely present that he does not allow himself to fall from the edge, and the same goes for the tantric woman in regards to what we call explosive orgasms. In tantric lovemaking the woman doesn't get the energy draining explosive orgasms. These are typically clitorisfocused orgasms that make her tighten and then release – explode – energy, and then afterwards leaves her tired, and with a feeling of: "Ah, that took off the pressure." A feeling of letting go of some energy, just like the man.

However, women do recharge much faster and have much more sexual energy than men, so therefore her discharge of energy is not as final as it is for the man. Often she will be able to continue and have more orgasms after a period of time. Still there is a feeling of less intensity and not as much energy as before. The tantric woman avoids orgasms that drain her energy, and instead she strives to reach the orgasms that do not explode, but that rather implode inwards and up, awakening her fully and actually filling her with more energy.

This is one of the major differences between the two types of orgasms – women can get many kind of orgasms, but we can place them into two different categories: the explosive orgasms and the implosive orgasms.

The explosive orgasm continuously builds up, until it reaches a clear point when it begins and then it ends again fast. It is just like a sneeze that you feel building up to the point of explosion, and then suddenly it is over. Maybe you sneeze again later, but it is not continuously, it is not like you can continue sneezing.

The implosive orgasms are more like a state of being that you enter, and can remain in infinitely or as long as you are able to handle the intense feeling. Very often the mind and the ego will tell you that you are about to lose yourself in this extremely expansive orgasm. It feels like you are losing your own normal personality i.e. suddenly you might feel that you have no name, no body, no thinking "What am I going to have for dinner tonight? Do I look good in this position?", or anything else. Everything that you normally identify with just suddenly dissolves and the woman experiencing this can just feel united with something much bigger than herself. This experience can be devastating for the ego, and therefore the ego will try to block it. That is why the mind will try to return to its normal state as soon as possible. But when we practice our ability to stay in this state of being, then we will be able to have a lot of orgasms that last for a very long time.

The tantric orgasm is a very different kind of orgasm. There is not the same focus on reaching an orgasm. It is something that might occur and when it does, it is very welcome, but there is nothing wrong if it doesn't. On the other hand, by practicing this ecstatic ability you begin to experience pleasure in everything you do during lovemaking. Earlier on you might have thought that the orgasm was the best part, but now it becomes the point from where you begin. This means that the pleasure and intensity change their character completely. Instead of building up more and more until we finally release, the state of orgasm instead becomes something we create and enter, expand and contain.

What is the difference between tantric massage and tantric lovemaking/sex?

Tantric lovemaking is a love meeting between two people who wish to unite at all levels. And through that union step out of their own ego by the power of the unity with someone else, and use this experience as a springboard to connect with something greater than themselves. It sounds so beautiful and right, but it can be so difficult. When we first begin, we are faced with our own desire, our own pleasure and our own inhibitions and conceptions of how it should all be: "What does she like? Am I good enough and am I hot enough"? All that which keeps us from being one with all that exists. We face both the conscious and unconscious aspects of ourselves.

The tantric massage gives us the perfect conditions to train these components that need to be in place before the lovemaking becomes magic. Some of the components that need training could be: to be able to receive touch, pleasure and love without always feeling that you have to give something in return and without being confronted with your own limitations in all kinds of ways. That could be actual traumas from the past, or maybe small misunderstandings about intimacy and sexuality, or for instance the feeling of: "I have to perform. What is he expecting from me? And should I moan, when I feel something because this is what I usually do?" All that can be used in the massage to find that space where we are able to feel what is real inside of ourselves, right here and now. Through a tantric massage you can actually return to your own natural sexuality.

If you begin to practice giving massages, then you can train the ability to give from the heart without expecting anything in return. Many people are used to getting something in return after giving a massage. The classic example is the man who says: "Do you want a massage, honey"? and then she knows what is expected to follow. And if she likes him, well, then that is great, because then he is offering to give her some pleasure before he gets his own pleasure, but there is still an expected outcome. So we must learn to fully give without expecting anything in return and be able to tune into someone, and to feel what goes on inside of her through our own hands, to feel what her soul needs, rather than what we are hoping for or wanting right now. We practice the ability to see beyond ourselves and to connect with another person.

That is why we recommend that the couples should learn the tantric massage, so they can learn how they can be together in a completely new intimate way and actually get to know each other much better than they have ever done before, even if they have been together for more than 20 years. In the massage they practice to receive 100% and to just feel themselves without doing anything for the other person. At the same time they practice being completely present for someone else and to give everything that they would wish to receive themselves. Most people are good at one of them, either giving or receiving, but rarely both.

But when we practice, and eventually master, both fully, then two people can merge, and what one of them wants will be exactly what the other one wish to give. Then there are no worries about giving and taking; no "now it´s my turn, now it´s your turn". In regular sex it very often happens that there is some pleasure, but then she also has to give something back, so he can get his blow job and his ejaculation, and then maybe he can give her an orgasm before they are done.

Through the tantric massage you can practice to go

beyond this pattern. But in order to do that, you must first practice the new patterns to the extreme. We must first practice to give fully and receive fully and not just practice something in between, there should be no half measures. When we are able to do this, then we can merge. During a massage a lot of couples will switch between giver and taker rather fast, before it starts to go deeper and get near a breakthrough and then start to have sex instead of continuing the massage. And then, exactly at the point where their love making could go even deeper, he ejaculates. Instead they should stay focused and go all the way in one direction at a time. Then next time they are together, they can go all the way in the other direction. To practice that ability is a part of the tantric massage, so you might say that the tantric massage is a way to practice tantric lovemaking.

Chapter 6: The man and the woman

Let's talk a bit more about man and woman. From a tantric perspective, what are the most significant differences between the sexes?

In the areas of eroticism, intimacy and love, both man and woman are capable of so much more than what they are already experiencing. We live in a society that is extremely limiting in regards to love and sexuality. Even if we think we are really free, we are still far away from realising our potential. In all pornography, for instance the porn you find on the internet, the male ejaculation is portrayed as the climax, the grand finale. This is extremely limiting for the masculine sexuality, because the man is actually able to separate the ejaculation from the orgasm, which enables him to have not just one, but several or even many orgasms without ejaculating during lovemaking. All this happens without him losing his energy, desire or erection which is so much more than what pornography portrays. Pornography says that we must aim for as much pleasure as possible until the sex is over, or until we reach our goal.

But instead of what is sometimes referred to as a "happy ending", tantra aims for "never ending happiness". Men can learn so much more about their own sexuality than what they have been brought up with. And when a man starts learning more, his sexuality will change and he will experience great changes in all areas of his life. He will feel it in his relations with women, his way of interacting with other people, his performance at work, his performance in sports, his way of being with his loved one, or the way he interacts with his own children. Everything will change completely, because now he has a strong force available to him, a power that is not wasted anymore because it is no longer released, because now he has learned to direct it inwards and upwards instead. And he will not feel like he is missing or sacrificing anything. Perhaps in the initial period of practice he will feel like he has to sacrifice the best part of his sex life, in order to learn something that is far, far better. The orgasms he will now be able to have will be bigger, longer and more powerful than the orgasms connected to an ejaculation, that last 5‑15 seconds at the most. He can now learn how to have much more intense orgasms lasting for minutes. He will be able to satisfy a woman much better and thereby gain confidence and a feeling of being at peace with his own masculinity, knowing that he is able to satisfy any kind of woman that he meets.

The female sexuality is basically much richer than the male sexuality. It is both greater and much more powerful than his.

This is not how our society portrays it?

No, and one of the reasons is that woman have much more sexual energy than men, but they are less aware of it.

The man has less sexual energy than the woman, but he is much more aware of it. That means that as soon as his desire is awakened, he is very attentive to it, in a "then we have to do something about it right"? kind of way, because this is the only thing on his mental screen now. The woman, on the other hand, has a completely different powerful energy, but she is very often not aware of it yet. If her sexuality awakens, then it becomes an enormous and completely unstoppable force of nature. When she learns how to use that energy and to awaken it fully, she will be able to profit enormously from her sexual energy. She can use it to awaken all kinds of qualities in herself as a woman and in all situations. As a mother, at work, in her art or whatever it may be. It comes rushing through her like a big and powerful river of sexual energy. The feminine primordial force will be empowering all her actions, and she will no longer feel that her actions are limited, dulled or inhibited, or that she is not adequate or good enough. Suddenly she has Mother Earth covering her back, and this can give her energy in a completely new way. The woman is naturally much more connected to the energy whereas the man is more connected to the consciousness which means that the woman can use this connection to empower her projects. If she is faced with a project, she can charge it with her energy and make it come alive, and if it is connected with a good plan, nothing keeps her from succeeding.

What are the man's challenges in regards to sexual energy and love?

The connection between sexuality and emotions is a

much bigger challenge for men than it is for women, and this is something many men need to work with. At first he needs to work on getting control of the sexual energy, and to master the energy better because then he can actually begin to send it up into his heart. It is difficult to lift up the energy after a daily ejaculation, because there is not much energy left to redirect to the upper chakras.

But some of the marvelous polarities between men and woman are that men are naturally more erotically open and more emotionally closed, and that women are more open at the emotional level and more closed at the erotic level.

When a man and a woman meet and fall in love, they open up wide to each other. And then all is well. She is erotically open and he is emotionally open. They feel that they match each other and might think that they have found the love of their life. After a couple of months the infatuation fades and they both fall back into their old natural patterns, and now suddenly she is no longer erotically open and he stops being emotionally open, and this is when the first conflicts appear. If instead they would learn how to approach each other in the best possible way, they would be able to avoid many problems and complications. A woman needs to be met in the heart, before she opens up sexually. Many men find that difficult to understand, just as many women have a have a hard time understanding that a man needs to be met sexually before he opens up his heart.

Let's say that husband and wife come home from work. They have both had busy days and are maybe a bit stressed. Then he says: "Hey baby", comes up behind her, and says:

"How about a quickie before dinner"? And then she replies: "No, I don't feel like it right now, maybe later. When you ask me in this way I have to say no, because this is how I feel right now". She is not open in her heart right now, so she is not ready. This makes him feel disappointed and rejected, because he was approaching her with the best that he has. And then it goes wrong. But at the same time, many women don't understand that making him sit down, asking him: "Honey, let's talk for a bit. How do you feel?" feels just as aggressive and intimidating to him, and that to him it feels like it would feel for her if he had just grabbed her yoni. The fact that she, without any kind of foreplay, wants to talk to him about his feelings makes him shut down. This is just as difficult for him, as it is for her to make love without foreplay and many women find it hard to understand and accept that he needs to be met sexually first. In a tantric massage the focus is on opening up the heart and making the erotic energy follow, making sure they go hand in hand. And once this is in sync, we add the spirituality. Sexuality, love and spirituality then become closely tied together, because when we put our hearts into our sexuality we truly open up to our spirituality and a greater force.

What sort of fears do men and women have about this?

The fear of letting go of the well known. To feel progress can actually be frightening.

The woman feels that the man has to prove his love, and only when he really shows his love will she dare to love him back. The moment he shuts off, she shuts off as well, and that is not real love. It is not unusual to hear people proclaim their mutual love and then they still end up hating each other a few years down the road. But then it was never actually real love. Love can not become hate, unless it was never love from the beginning. The feeling they thought was love was actually expectations about how things should be. Only our expectations can give us this kind of anger, disappointment and hurt. Love itself has no expectations, and therefore it cannot be disappointed, hurt or sad. Love just wants to love. It is our own expectations of the results of this love that make us feel disappointment. In tantra we work on being present in the love we feel without building up a lot of expectations, or dragging our personal history into the love. We try to let go of everything that has happened, been said or done, and instead say: "In this moment it is my wish to love you as much as possible. To love you just as you are right now, and not expect anything of you that is based upon what you have done before."

And when it comes to love we all want it so badly, yet it is so difficult. Just as it is with sexual experiences, we all want it but it can be so very difficult to achieve.

This often happens because we communicate in such different ways. Men and woman communicate differently. Most men feel that they should not say anything unless they really mean it. A man's word is his word, something you can build upon and trust. And when it comes to feelings, he knows very well that he may not feel the same way tomorrow and therefore he might feel a strong pressure when he is asked to express his emotions. It can be very difficult to say "I love you" – he might mean it at the moment, but feels that it has to be objectively true in order for him to speak it. He needs to believe that he will still feel this way for at least a year or two if he is to speak these words. Knowing that his feelings might change significantly can make it difficult for him to put them into words.

The woman on the other hand, will express how she feels right now. Therefore it might be easier for her to say: "I love you" right now, if that is what she feels right now. And therefore it is also easier for her to say: "I hate you" the day after, or: "Leave me alone, I don't want to see you anymore". This can feel very confusing and upsetting for the man, because then he feels that he cannot trust her. She will say one thing today and another tomorrow, and this is not something a man feels he can trust. But the woman has spoken the truth in both instances, she has expressed her true feelings in the moment. This is just very different from the male concept of truth, which is more like: "When I say something it must be objectively true, otherwise I'm a liar". This difference can of course cause many complications.

And then, if he finally tells her that he loves her, he feels that he doesn't have to tell her again, unless something changes, because he already told her. However, she would like to hear it again and again, because she wants him to confirm that this is how he still feels about her.

Besides working on improving the communication, we should also use the active love in order to return to our own centre and thereby find our balance. The principle of active love is about action, expressing our love, turning love into action like words and behaviour, helping others without waiting for the love to be returned.

In tantra we believe that the woman leads the way. The woman intuitively understands that sexuality can be both beautiful and elevated, and that it can awaken them both spiritually. Therefore it is the woman who needs to awaken the man; and most often he is not a man with a tantric background who is all ready to meet her new needs. It is most likely a man, or several men, with the potential to be awakened by her guidance, courage and patience.

Part of woman's nature is to be the initiating woman. This means a woman who is capable of awakening the man, the one, who can lead him into sensuality and intimacy in a completely new way, who doesn't allow him to get caught in his instinctive urges and who just lifts him up and awakens him to completely new dimensions. This woman can be found within all women. But she is most often restricted by the fear of getting hurt or the tendency to let her emotional life take over and make him responsible for her wellbeing, believing that it is his responsibility to make her happy. If she believes that, then she will remain unhappy. She will remain unhappy even with the best man if she expects him to make her happy. If she can find her own happiness within herself, she can then become a fantastic inspiration for both men and women, who can be inspired by her way of loving, her way of living and everything that she touches.

When she is awakened she has to dare to lift the energy

higher and this requires that she is willing to lift herself up to a new level, where she can gain a new perspective on herself, her life and her way of interacting with men.

How do men and woman approach a tantric massage differently?

When men come to visit the Tantra Temple to get a massage, the often have a feeling of "WOW, here is a fantastic, tantric, sensual, beautiful woman who gives me this amazing massage, who makes me feel more like a man than I have ever felt before, who shows me new sides of myself and opens up new possibilities for what I can do and what I am capable of". He will be ready to follow this kind of woman and learn more from her, and this is the level that women should aspire to reach. He feels that this is an initiating woman, who helps him to become a better version of himself. When a woman, who is just slightly awakened, meets a man she should choose to lift herself up to this level and say: "I do not want superficial sex anymore from now on I only want uplifting and beautiful erotic experiences". When a man experiences this, he would drop would long to follow her into this universe. But if he tries to drag her down to the level of superficial sex again, and she is willing to compromise, then she will later have to find her way back to herself and lift herself up once more.

Many women, who come for tantra massage, has to practice clearing themselves of the role they often take on in erotic situations. Some women are raised to be "the nice girl", and for some it is the opposite. We might call her: "the porn queen", the woman who begins to moan and scream, as soon as she gets tickled on the neck. She is not true to herself, she is just playing a role. And the nice girl, the one who suppresses her emotions and needs, and who never shows the world how she really feels, she is also playing a role and therefore not true to her nature.

In a tantric massage the woman is invited to give herself permission to feel what is really going on, how she really feels, and to just express that. It might come out "wrong" in the beginning, and not at all the way she wants to express it. But the more she practices , the closer she will get to letting go of other people's expectations. Her boyfriend might have some expectations of her, of how she should be but the tantra masseur doesn't have any expectations of how she should behave or react, or how the massage should unfold for her. She can just relax completely and feel the energy move inside her.

The more she lets herself relax, the more she allows the energy to move her body, instead of her mind controlling what her body does. When she does this, when she really lets go, then her movements will become more fluid, like waves. The energy knows what to do, so when she permits the energy to move her body, it will do so in a way that helps the energy flow freely.

For many women this is an entirely new experience, because they are so used to blocking the energy by tightening up and being wrapped up in their thoughts of how it should be. Many women discover new qualities in themselves as well as new dimensions of the energy. She might feel a very powerful energy buzzing and twirling everywhere, making her feel that she is growing and expanding and becoming much larger than her physical body. This is all very basic in tantra, but many people have never experienced something like this before, because they are stuck in old habits and old ideas of how things should be.

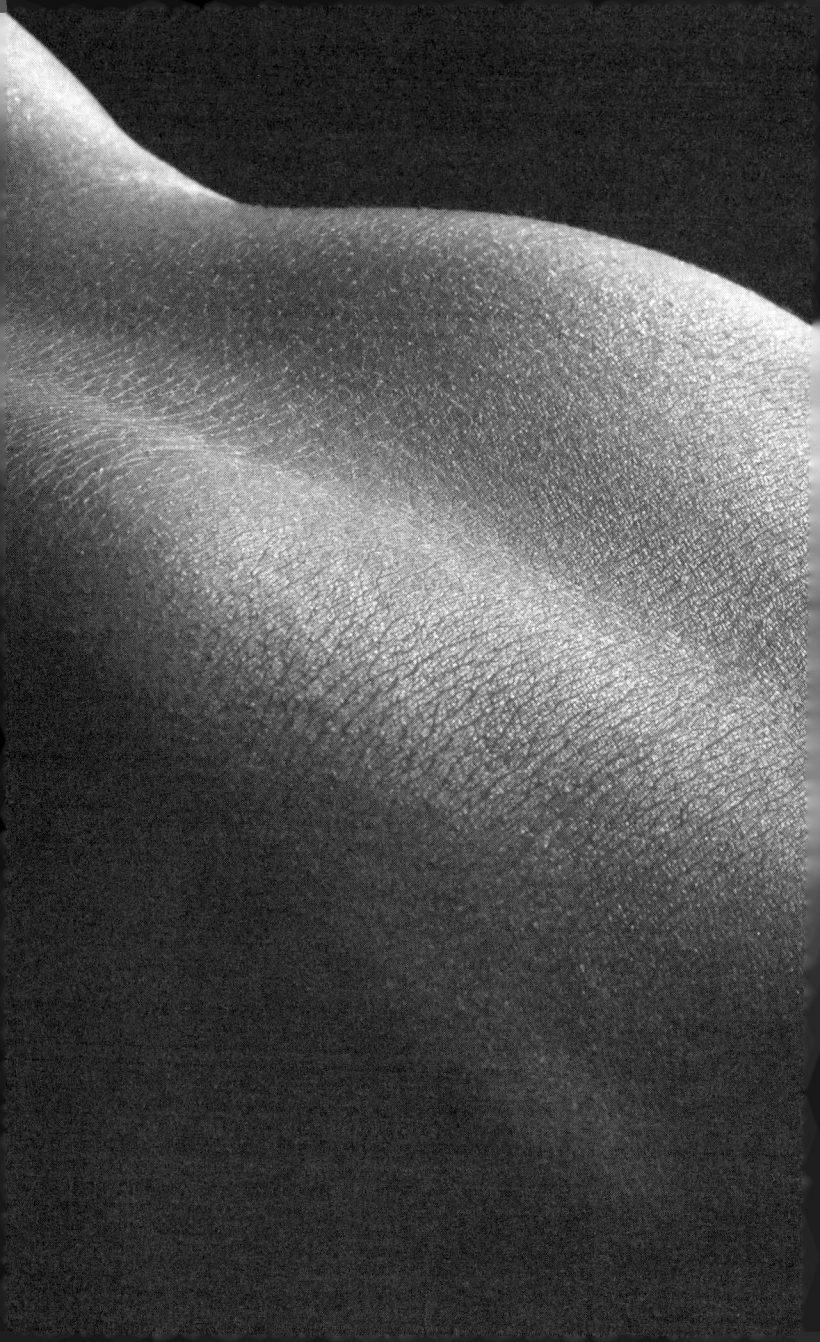

Chapter 7:
You, me and tantra

What about when tantra is about two people?

We began by defining the four cornerstones of tantra. We talked about polarity, energy, love and transfiguration, and how to practice all of these in a profound way in a loving relationship with another human being. Love unfolds itself the most, when we love someone. Transfiguration works better when we have someone in whom we see the divine. Polarity works better when we have someone to polarise, and sexual continence works better when we practice it. Of course we can also choose to be abstinent, that is also a possibility. However, it is much more effective when we manifest our sexual energy.

Tantric relationships are different from traditional relationships. If you are in a traditional relationship, there are still a number of tantric techniques, based upon the four cornerstones of tantra, that you can use to improve your relationship.

Polarity

This means that energy arises from polarity, and energy arises from differences. We recognise this principle from electricity, where we have a positive pole and a negative pole and this creates the voltage. We also know this from magnets, where the north pole and the south pole attract each other. In a tantric relationship you will naturally choose to work with polarity in a conscious way. Just as we also work with many other aspects at a highly conscious level. It is much more than just: "Are we feeling good, and if we feel good, is it good enough? And if we are not feeling good, then we should do something to make it better."

In a tantric relationship you will continuously make sure that you are moving in the right direction. Even if you are feeling better than ever. You will quite quickly notice if something is going wrong and not hesitate to correct it, even long before you reach the point where one of you say: "Baby, we need to talk." You will always be keeping a finger on the pulse of the relationship to check if the polarity and thus attraction, is still there. You will automatically check to see if you are doing something that makes the polarity and attraction fade, and how you can change it, not in order to awaken a dying flame, but in order to constantly feed the fire and keep it alive

In tantra the man practices his masculine qualities and the woman practices her feminine qualities in order to awaken more polarity. The point is, that the more you work with your own natural polarity, the more you will be the opposite pole. A very masculine man will naturally attract a very feminine woman and in that meeting lots of energy will be created, much more than in the case of a man and a woman, who are very much alike, and therefore not creating a lot of polarity.

Many modern couples do not give themselves and their relationship the best conditions. If you spend a lot of disconnected time together, the attraction will naturally fade. Meaning that the more time you spend together, without really doing anything together, but just being together in each your separate worlds, the more you will undermine the attraction. In tantra we actually encourage that the meeting between the lovers becomes a very intense encounter. And then we encourage separation for a while, to be followed by another intense meeting, again followed by separation. The length of the meetings and the separation periods can vary from one relationship to the other. For some, the separation might last much longer than the meeting, and for others it might be the other way around. Most importantly you have to be attentive to when you should be together and when it is time to separate. This way of being together then becomes a cycle, just as anything else in life, like the way we breathe in and breathe out. Everything has its own cycle. Like night and day. We have the polarity of the man and the woman. Being together is like breathing in one another. Inhaling the amazing and nurturing energy arising from the connection. But we must also remember to breathe out. At the beginning of relationships many people believe that they can just keep breathing each other in, because it feels so good. But it is not possible. At some point one of them will say: "I have had enough and I need a break", but the other person might not understand why, because he or she has not yet reached the point of suffocation.

When a tantric relationship is at its best you will often choose to separate for a while. Just when both lovers think it is fantastic, right then it is actually time to polarise again. Because by separating while everything is really good, you immediately begin to long for one another. In this way you create a condition where you are only together when you have a great desire to be together.

Recognising that this is the way polarisation works helps many couples find a way of both being together and also being separated. A lot of relationships don't have space for that. The couple shares an apartment or a house that provides what they need as a couple, however they have to find somewhere else or even hide if they want to separate a bit. Many people share the romantic idea of the perfect family spending all their time together, or a relationship where you spend as much time together as possible when not at work. You eat together, sleep together, watch TV together and have sex together. This means that if one partner feels he or she needs some space, then the other partner immediately thinks something is wrong. Instead, it would make much more sense to develop a relationship where there is space both to be together and also to be on your own.

Energy

Sexual continence, meaning the ability to master our own sexual energy, is a wonderful practice in a relationship. It is the ongoing wish to improve your ability to master this energy. Women are naturally better skilled at this than men, not only in regards to premature orgasms, but women are also much better at moving their sexual energy. It is usually much more difficult for the man, which is why the woman is said to lead the man at the intimate level. She has a natural ability to connect the sexual energy to a higher spiritual level.

She is equipped with the innate knowledge that sexuality can be more beautiful and glorious than just the instinctive gratification of desire.

In tantra the woman leads the way into intimacy. It is also she who helps him practice mastering his sexual energy. In the beginning she will lead the way and help him develop. Once he has become really good, it is actually he who helps her the last steps of the way. Then he can help her lift their sexual energy, and not just get lost in pleasure. In the beginning, when the man easily gets lost in pleasure, it is difficult for the woman to understand his lack of control, because she has most often not yet experienced much pleasure herself. But once he has become a super lover, it is she who easily gets lost in pleasure, because he is able to give her hours of continuous orgasms. Then it becomes his responsibility to lift their sexual energy to the highest possible level.

Love

Love should be what brings and keeps us together. Surely love is the starting point of many relationships, but then they start building all kind of things on top of the love. In the beginning there is a lot of sexual attraction, not to be confused with love. Soon the lovers begin to build a life together on top of this attraction, and they may even move in together. They start to share the same friends, maybe they buy a house together, a car, maybe they even have children together. They add a lot of things on top of the love that isn't love. They keep adding so much that eventually the structure will still stand, even if the love is removed. From the outside it will still appear to be a relationship.

Now it is primarily all the practical stuff that keeps them together. Many people feel that when they have children, they forget to be man and woman, and they just become mom and dad instead. Then, around 15 years later when the children are teenagers, the couple visit the Tantra Temple, and then they say: "We have forgotten how to be together. We now finally have the time and opportunity to be together, but we don't know how"? They need to find themselves and each other again, because the eroticism and intimacy was forgotten over the years. They had no space to make love, which is very unfortunate since lovemaking is the best way to express love.

In a tantric relationship, love is always the first priority. Love is what brought us together, what holds us together, and the reason why we still want to be together. We do not allow anything to come between us and love. Meaning that if we realise that part of what binds us together or that some of our habits are not based on love, then we need to clear it up. The tantric couple will constantly aim to remove all unconscious habits, and they will always return to love and to the questions: "How does our love feel? Do we love each other"? Or if we experience that the love is fading, we ask ourselves: "What can we do about it? How can we awaken even more love for each other"?

A truly loving relationship can be stripped from all habits, social contexts and material possessions, and the lovers can be placed on a desolate island, and they would still have a deep and beautiful relationship.

When love fades away, many couples remain together without really doing anything about it. They don't feel good about being together anymore, but they still stay together because divorce is too difficult. They begin asking whether they can afford the divorce, if they can find a new place to live, and so on. Suddenly they recognise all the things that are keeping them together. Love dies when the glue in the relationships is all the outer things.

Putting love into words and actions awaken the heart. You can reactivate the love by giving love instead of waiting to feel love. For instance you can send short messages, declarations of love, gifts, attention, touch or whatever it may be, with the sole purpose and desire to make your loved one as happy as possible.

If you are with someone who feels the same way, it becomes a real winwin situation, where both lovers want the other one to be as happy as possible at all times. Rather than two people with a selfcentered focus on receiving a certain measure of pleasure and happiness from the relationship before they are willing to invest themselves in it. This latter attitude could give thoughts like: "I don't want to invest my love in this person anymore, because he or she doesn't live up to my expectations.

Transfiguration

Transfiguration is also an essential element of the tantric relationship. This is the ability to see the beauty and divinity in the other person, recognise their potential and help them cultivate it. Sometimes you will discover qualities that this person is not aware of yet, and thereby you can help him or her awaken and cultivate them.

The fusion

Tantra seeks to teach people, how they can not only get the best out of their sexuality, but actually lift the sexual experience to levels that are much higher than just sex. That tantric sexuality is an expression of love, and that the fusion connects us to something much greater than ourselves.

In the tantric relationship the lovers lift and support each other. They use each other as a mirror, they are able to learn and evolve much faster than if they were alone. In tantra we believe that everything is created out of polarity, plus and minus, the masculine and the feminine, Shiva and Shakti. We have the consciousness and the energy. The man and the woman become human manifestations of Shiva and Shakti. They will have much more energy available, if they manage to build up the polarity and use the energy actively. If they both focus on the same goal or the same thing, they have much more energy available and they will therefore be able to achieve more. In the spiritual relationship, there is a great aspiration to lift each other up, and an innate knowledge that they can both evolve significantly. The lovers are searching for transformation, and they are actively striving to develop themselves more. They are ready to accept that the other person will not remain the same as he or she was the day before. A more traditional relationship will focus more on maintaining status quo and is more likely to hold on to how it was yesterday. When things go wrong, they try to go back to the good old days and the beginning of their relationship.

Tantra is about accepting constant transformation in ourselves, the other person and our surroundings. In a tantric relationship you will never hear your beloved say: "You usually do like this….." You are always considered to be a completely unlimited and divine individual.

If one of you forgets that this is what you are, then your beloved will remind you: "Do not forget that you are a completely unlimited and divine being. You have just gotten caught up in an emotional mess". You both realise that it the current drama is quite insignificant in the big scheme of it all, and you help each other remain focused on your spiritual development.

The lovemaking

In tantric lovemaking, all five senses are fully and completely engaged. And so they are during regular lovemaking as well. That is one of the reasons why lovemaking is so intense. But in tantric lovemaking you strive to become fully aware of all the sensations. Lovemaking is one of the most intense experiences we can have as humans. Not only because the sexual energy is one of the strongest energies, but also because it is an activity involving all five senses. When we make love, we smell one another, taste one another, see one another, feel one another and listen to one another.

If you removed even one of the senses it would be a completely different experience, and if you removed even more senses, it would be a very poor experience. When I say "remove", I mean with the lack of focus. Attempting to make love without using your sense of smell, or with the lights out, can be a stimulating experience for some, forcing them to focus on the other senses. But if not wanting to see what goes on is the general approach, then we are keeping ourselves from being present. Then the experience is subject to our mental filter and becomes dominated by our expectations and fears based upon prior experiences.

In the tantric lovemaking you consciously work with the intense awakening of the senses, knowing that it helps us to be present in the moment.

Tantric lovemaking might very well begin with a ritual of arousing the senses. During traditional foreplay you kiss a little, touch a little, lick a little and then you start. Instead we might begin by being fully present with one sense at a time. We might take the time to smell each other in different places. How does the mouth smell? the armpits? the genitals? The hair? etc. There are so many different smells all over the body, and we let ourselves fill up with the experiences from that sense. Afterwards we deeply enter the sense of taste by tasting each other all over. Followed by the rest of our senses, one by one. Once you have been through them all, and have taken the other fully in, as he/she has done with you, then you are already close to being fully fused. When you then introduce the lingam into the yoni, and the actual fusion happens, you are already fully open towards one another in all your complexity.

Let's talk tantra sex or...?

I would rather call it tantric lovemaking, because the word "lovemaking" makes me think of it as two people who love each other, and who wish to connect to one another. To me sex is an expression of a need that wants to be gratified, in the same… way that the need to drink, sleep and eat are all needs that seek gratification. The only difference is that sex is a need we meet together with another person. But the term making love goes so much deeper into the wish of wanting to love someone so much that you are able to fuse together; able to unite with one another. I would like to make these terms clear right from the beginning of this talk.

When we begin to talk about how tantric lovemaking differs from regular sex, we come right back to the four cornerstones of tantra. One of them is that if you want to call it tantric lovemaking, there has to be a deep love between the two lovers, and when I say two it actually doesn't need to be two. Theoretically it can be a situation where a person is making love to him/herself, or many people making love together. But no matter what, there has to be a deep love. There has to be love for yourself, and love for the one or ones you are making love with. Many people think that tantra is all about group sex. But in reality, an erotic tantric encounter involving more than two people is rather difficult, because it requires you to have a deep feeling of love for everyone in the group.

The love is essential in order to call it tantric lovemaking. In addition, the ability to control and master the sexual energy what we call sexual continence is essential if you want to call it tantric lovemaking. Just as it is absolutely essential that the sexual energy is awakened and used for the higher purpose of awakening other aspects of ourselves and the higher chakras. Transfiguration is essential as well. This is our ability to see beyond the immediate, to see a greater force, and the divinity in the experience, and how the woman and man through their union can become universal archetypes.

It is important for both the man and the woman with a long foreplay in tantric lovemaking. The woman needs time to really open up, relax and become completely receptive, especially in her pelvis, so that she can reach the point where every cell in her body yearns to be penetrated. This is the point where she is so open that she longs to be full of him instead of just being wet enough for penetration, as it often goes in normal sex.

For the man the long foreplay is important because it can help him awaken the energy at a pace that allows him to stay in control and master the energy. In this way he does not ejaculate quickly, lose control of himself, or get caught in the more beastly and instinctual force, where he would lose contact with her and instead become absorbed with himself and his own pleasure. The long foreplay helps him become much more conscious about the energy, and it helps him awakening it at a pace that allows him to master it, and thereby it becomes much easier for him to make love for a long time. If the foreplay is short and straight on, it is much more difficult for him to control the energy.

This does not mean that tantric lovemaking goes on for hours every time. One can easily imagine a tantric "quickie", taking only 20 to 30 minutes. It is always a question of how much time you have, and how much time you have set aside for it. Some might think it has to last for hours every time, but it does not. Instead it requires that you prioritize your sexuality and that you sincerely wish to become a better lover and learn how to use the energy for a higher purpose. This means that once in a while you need to set aside proper time for it.

Imagine a person, who wants to excel at sport, saying: "I only want to practice when I am in the mood for it". His coach would most likely say: "Fine, you do that. But then I am not able to help you".

Pleasure and sexuality are a part of the practice in tantra and this means that we practice regularly. Pleasure almost becomes the rule; that we have to practice at least twice a week on getting bigger and better orgasms. If you only practice when you feel desire, you will never learn how to consciously awaken this desire. If we don't learn to awaken desire consciously, we will be controlled by the rise and fall of the desire and the idea that: "We will not make love until we feel the desire, and then we will only do it if we accidentally both feel it at the same time". With help of tantric techniques you become able to awaken the desire and energy at will. This means that you can plan ahead and say "Let's meet

Saturday and spend four hours together", and then you begin to build up to this day, so that the energy will be at the highest when the meeting happens. You might do some exercises in the days before, or on that particular day, to help the energy be at its highest; both your vital energy, sexual energy and emotional energy. This is a conscious way of working with energy, instead of just unconsciously waiting for a peak in the energies, and then enjoying them for the fun of it?.

In tantric lovemaking we work consciously with the energy, and we work with the principle that whatever we focus on, when the energy is the most powerful, is where this energy will go. If you roll over on the other side, and fall asleep right after making love, you direct the energy to sleeping, thus investing it in being unconscious. When that happens you do not use the energy consciously, and instead you give it to whatever you are dreaming about. If you jump out of the bed and begin reading the news on Facebook, or start watching television, then that is where your energy goes.

If you, on the other hand, do something together after the lovemaking, then this is what the energy will empower. If for instance you make a meditation, where you focus in your heart and on the love you have for one another right after your lovemaking, then you will strengthen the love. If you start working on your art, you are actually able to actively channel your energy into it. If you begin your spiritual practice afterwards, and choose to do yoga, well, then this is where the energy flows. This is what many Tantrics choose to do. They use the sexual energy for their spiritual journey, for their spiritual development. They use it when it is most powerful, right after they have made love for a long time, and have awakened more of the spiritual energy. The spiritual practice you do in that moment has so much more power than "just" a regular yoga practice, because of the extra energy you possess. The way you choose to use the energy afterwards is yet another thing that differentiates tantric lovemaking from traditional sex.

Does it do a couple good to take a break from being sexually active, and then start up again fresh?

For many people starting out with tantra, it would help a lot to completely reboot and clear the hard disk from all that they have learned about sexuality, and then start all over. Even if you have been in the same relationship for 10‑20 years, and have had a good sex life, it is still good to let go of everything that you have learned, and begin to get to know one another all over.

In a modern relationship it is not always that easy to pull out the plug completely. But naturally it is possible to stop making love for a while and instead build up a new form of intimacy, closeness and strong desire to unite rather than just responding to desire and the wish to "take off the edges". If you really want to master the sexual energy, you have to go beyond the need to take off the edges, and instead awaken the energy and make it flow so freely that you don't feel any pressure. There are two ways to take relieve the pressure: One is to release the energy [through ejaculation or explosive orgasm], and the other one is to lift the energy. If you would really like to get the energy flowing, it can be a good idea not to make love for a period of time, anywhere from 1 to 3 months, and instead practice new forms of intimacy and closeness, deep eye contact, touch and massage. Not just to give each other pleasure, but to connect through conscious touch. To use the touch as a means to feel what goes on inside your beloved. After that, you can gradually begin to make love again, but in a completely different way, where you give it high priority in life, making it something much more beautiful and exalted, something you would wish to set time aside for.

You have to create new conditions and frames for this new way of making love. It is important to take the lovemaking out of the everyday patterns; make sure the kids are taken care of, that the phones and TV are turned off and that the computer is gone and out of sight, so that it doesn't interfere. Ask your beloved to take a long warm bath, put on candles and good music, and make sure the room smells nice and that all the senses are met with beautiful sensations. There has to be something for the sense of smell, sense of taste, sense of sight, sense of touch and sense of hearing. It has to be warm in the room. It is no good if it is cold. It needs to be so warm that you can be naked together without having to be under the covers. Then you take your beloved by the hand and bring him or her into the room, shut the door and say: "Now it is just the two of us. We can talk about our feelings towards one another, but we cannot talk about the kids, the job, the house, shopping or anything practical. Now it is just about our love for each other. Now we are cultivating our love life and not our practical life". You can then choose from a wide range of techniques, such as sensual massage, meditating together, gazing deeply into each other's eyes, feeling each other's love, feeling each other's hearts and exploring each other's erogenous zones.

It is a really good idea to find information about the different erogenous zones of the female and male body, and then start exploring. Experiment with touching each other in different ways and places around the body, and to find out together how to best awaken each other sexually. It is all about practicing and playing and getting to know your beloved as much as possible. Next time you switch, instead of having the attitude of: "I have given you some, now it is my turn to get some". Take it one encounter at a time, and forget about bartering.

Women are naturally multiorgasmic and able to have many different orgasms. They can be aroused in different ways, by different stimulation, and in different places, all over the body. Some women can have orgasms just by stimulation of the breasts, and some women can have orgasms if you suck her big toe long enough. The ability is there, the women is completely fantastic... she is unlimited.

Is the female sexuality more powerful than the male?

Yes, it is, but many people think the opposite, because the man appears to have more desire. This is so even though he has less energy than the woman because he is much more aware of what he has than the woman is... She is unaware of the volcano she is sitting on. Once her energy begins to awaken, it is extremely powerful, but she is not as aware of it. The man, on the other hand, is very aware of his sexual energy, and as soon as his lingam moves, he asks himself: "What can I do with this energy"?

The female sexuality is in a way far richer than the male, but that does not mean that the male sexuality is poor. The man is able to learn how to have multiple orgasms without ejaculation and this enables him to have many orgasms in a row. He can practice his ability to have orgasms that last longer and longer, and to be in a orgasmic state of being for several minutes, or more.

The woman is much more nuanced. She can have many various and distinct kinds of orgasms.

A wonderful practice in a relationship can be if the man says: "How about we try to see what kinds of different orgasms you can have"? This practice is so good, because even if the woman hears that she is able to have different kinds of orgasms, it can be quite difficult for her to ask the man: "How about we try to explore how many kinds of orgasms I can have"? The initiative has to come from the man. His curiosity to help her get to know herself better will naturally polarise and awaken her.

This is especially important during the period where they are learning sexual continence, and where he is training how to last longer and avoid ejaculation. During this period of time, when he is not quite continent yet, and the woman doesn't feel fully satisfied, it helps make their relationship more even, since she feels that he wants to do his best for her. If he is balancing on the edge of what is too much pleasure for him during their lovemaking, this can be a period where she is not fully satisfied in their lovemaking. She has to be very patient in this training period, because after they have made love for a little while, it will become too much for him and they will need to stop for a little while, and then start again. It would be a good challenge for him to learn how to stimulate the woman in various ways, so he can "trigger" all kinds of different orgasms, and thereby expand her erotic capability, just as he is in the middle of expanding his erotic capability.

One hint about how he can give a woman more pleasure and bring her into ecstasy is that he should stimulate at least 3 primary erogenous zones at once.

That means that he might kiss her, stimulate one or both her nipples and her clitoris, or that his lingam stimulates her gspot, while he is stimulating her clitoris and anus at the same time. There are numerous combinations and ways to stimulate.

It doesn't have to be only the primary erogenous zones. Many women become very frustrated that the foreplay is either too short or too targeted. It seems as if he is following a script, and based upon her reactions, he makes his next move, because this is what he is used to.

First and foremost it is important that he gives her a good foreplay with the sincere wish to awaken her fully, and not just in order to press some buttons to awaken just enough energy to get her excited. But it is also important that the foreplay does not stop when the lovemaking begins. She must be touched, moved around, massaged and kissed all over while they make love. The foreplay is not just something you do to build up so you can enter, and then you only stimulate inside the yoni with the lingam. The woman needs to be kissed, touched, and stimulated all over all the time, to bring her to ecstasy, instead of just making her ready to be penetrated.

When you adapt this attitude towards sexuality, then you are able to create situations that lift you up and help you grow. You continue to see new and more profound perspectives and you recognize that the woman is unlimited. And right after she has just had the most intense orgasm of her life, she is still ready for more, she is still ready to take it one step further. It can be really frustrating for the lazy man, because he might think that she is happy now that he has become a better lover. Her sex life might be better than before, but she is able to take it much further, and she cannot just settle with a certain level and be happy there. However, if you are both willing to grow together, you have the opportunity to lift your sexuality to a much higher level than the merely instinctive. This is a level where it is not about taking the edge off, but about using sexuality to raise each other to a higher level, and make a fusion possible. When two people unite and become one greater entity, or when they experience a state of androgyny that neutralises the differences between the masculine and feminine, they discover divinity, and together they become divine.

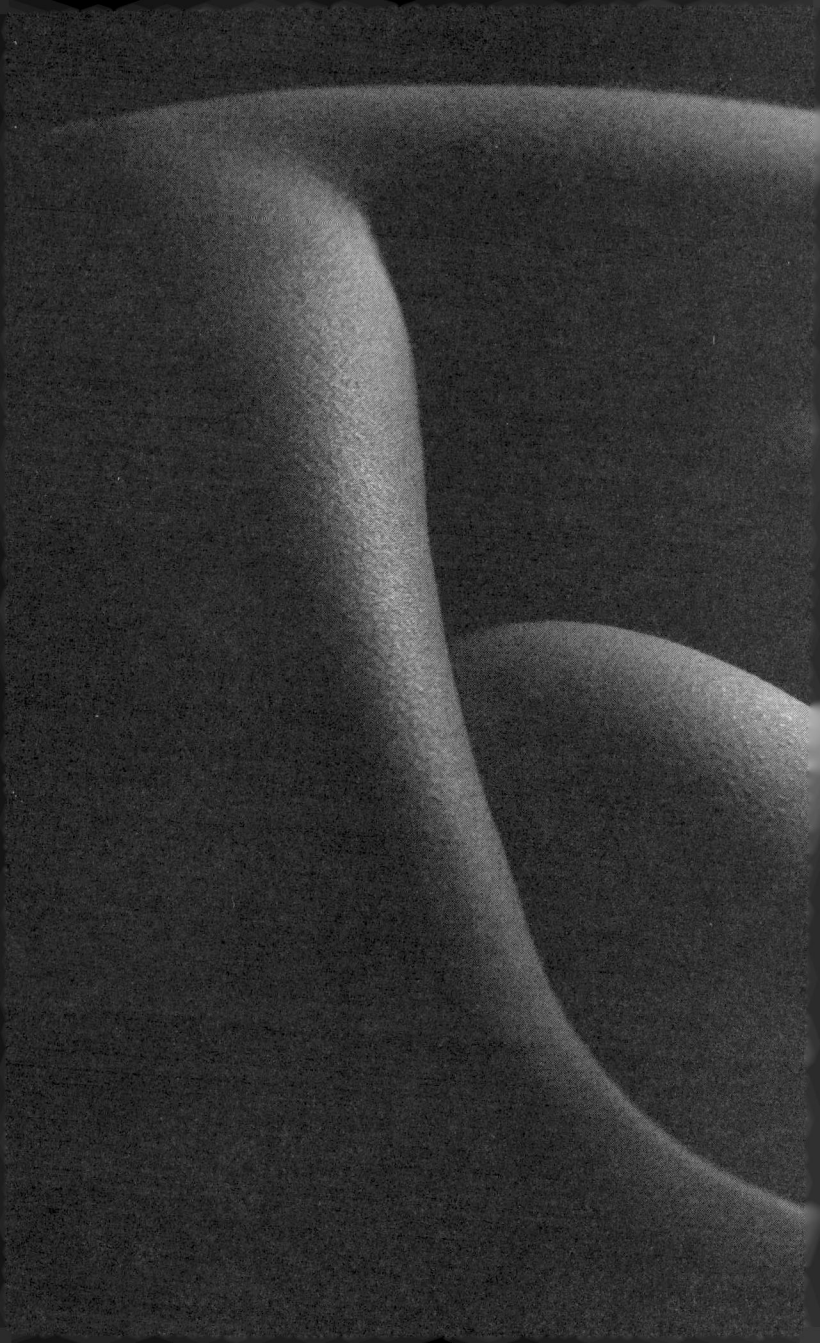

Chapter 8: Tantra's goal & wrapping up

Does tantra have a goal?

Tantra is a spiritual path, and like all other authentic spiritual paths, the goal is to recognise our own divine, and to reveal the divine spark inside of ourselves that is normally hidden from us in our daily lives. If tantra has a goal, that would be it. The goal is not to become the perfect lover, having better sex and experiencing amazing orgasms, healing your traumas or becoming a better person. These can be considered great milestones or natural steps along the way that leads to a revelation of our supreme Self. We are already at the goal we are aiming for. We have just forgotten this. The goal is to recognise that we already have it all within. We are all naturally moving towards this realisation. Tantra and other spiritual paths just speed up the process and have a higher awareness of what is blocking us. During this process many people recognise: "I am limited by my thoughts and my mind. My mind tries to tell me that I am limited to this body and this brain, these thoughts and feelings. My mind tries to limit me by making me believe that I will not live forever and that life ends when my body dies".

From there I can begin to work on my mind and I can learn new methods to quiet the mind and turn off the thoughts. This is where yoga comes in as an important method. "Yoga" means the union of the individual consciousness and the cosmic consciousness, and it helps us realise that we are a part of it all.

Full enlightenment will occur at some point, but actually it happens all the time. We experience glimpses of enlightenment all the time. They are just generally so short that we are not able to become aware of them. However, all spiritual practices have the purpose to expand these glimpses until they are long and strong enough so that we can recall these states, when we return to our normal state. The first glimpse of enlightenment can be a life changing landmark in a person's life, because in your normal conscious state you will then be able to remember that you have seen a glimpse of eternity. The purpose of the spiritual practice is to cleanse your structure and prepare for that experience to occur, because if you are not ready, you cannot apply it. Otherwise it can actually make people feel more disconnected. If this happens, they can become really discouraged and think: "Meditation is just not for me". If your perception is very restricted, it will not be able to cope with glimpses of eternity, and instead it can make you really sick.

A lot of people hang trophies on their wall of spirituality, showing the world what kind of experiences they have had. In tantra we do not work with trophies, but rather with making the spiritual experiences our own. Meaning that if we have been in a very intense spiritual state, it only matters if we are able to return to that state of consciousness by ourselves at will.

It is quite common for people who meditate to experience many fascinating things, which they can then later write about, for instance feelings and visions they have had. Tantra recognises the impact of the experience and that it is a sign that something higher is possible. The object is to refrain from just taking a picture of that state of being to hang on your wall, and then going out to find a new experience. The point is to willfully return to the state and then gradually recognise what unlimited beings we are.

All this sounds immensely beautiful and maybe as a goal not everyone can relate to. But can you make a conclusion, something that relates to everybody? You just said that tantra is for everybody?

Yes, and thank you for bringing it up, because tantra IS for everybody. And as I mentioned earlier, it begins just where you are right now. There is no right nor wrong goal in tantra. But if we want to talk about the supreme goal, then it would be to recognise our true spiritual nature and acknowledge the spark of divinity, which we all carry inside of us. To acknowledge that we are eternal and infinite beings, and that we are not limited by our conceptions of time and space.

It is therefore important to point out that all the goals you started out with are what you need to focus on. Whether it is to heal yourself, have a better sex life, a better relationship, a better sense of yourself or whatever it may be. Once you have reached that goal, new horizons will open, and new possibilities will develop. Every step, every recognition is a seed, that has been planted and will sprout and grow in whatever direction you fertilize it, and tantra offers you all possibilities for growth.

At the same time it is important to recognise that tantra only becomes alive through practice and awareness. I hope that everyone, who has picked up this book, feel better equipped to take the first step into practicing tantra in the form of tantric massage, tantric yoga or tantric lovemaking. Or if you already know tantra well – that you have been assured or have expanded your awareness of tantra.

In conclusion I would just like to say: take the leap, embrace it and remember that all journeys are different, and there is no limits in tantra. Listen to your heart. It has all the answers to how you can create the life that is waiting for you.

> Today I choose love
> Today I choose to love the others
> Before they love me

About the Tantra Temple

The Tantra Temple was founded in 2006 in Copenhagen, Denmark.

The initiative came from a group of tantric initiates, who had been practicing and teaching tantra for a number of years, and who had experienced profound transformation of their own lives. They felt that their experiences with consciousness, energy and love were so essential and profound that they could not just keep this knowledge to themselves – they had to find a way to share this understanding with others.

In tantra there is an ancient tradition for passing on knowledge, love, energy and even higher states of consciousness to others through direct initiation. Nowadays tantric massage proves to be a very efficient method to show people directly that they are hiding a much greater potential than they are aware of.

With branches spread across Europe and an international Tantra Massage Education the Tantra Temple has now become one of the leading tantric temples in the world.

Read more at www.tantra-temple.com

About Let's Talk serien

The Let's Talk book is a book series of vital books on different subjects. Every subject is carefully selected with the intent of bringing it towards a comprehensive level, enfolding the reader into the world of the subject matter. Every book has a tight structure and the people who have been chosen to talk about their field of expertise are highly competent. The vision is to create a space for new ideas to develop and to spark new thoughts in the reader, making a positive difference in the realization of their human potential.